SPIRITUAL
SEX

SPIRITUAL
SEX

Michelle Pauli

Illustrated by Alan Adler

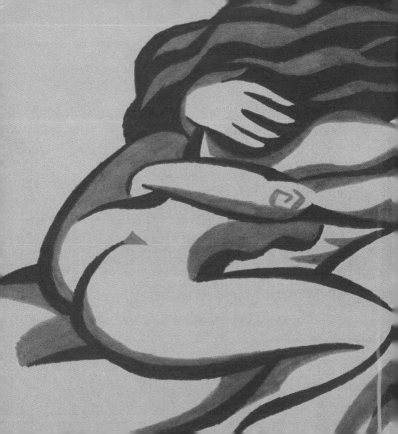

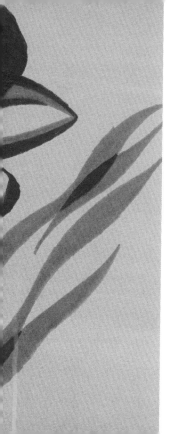

Contents

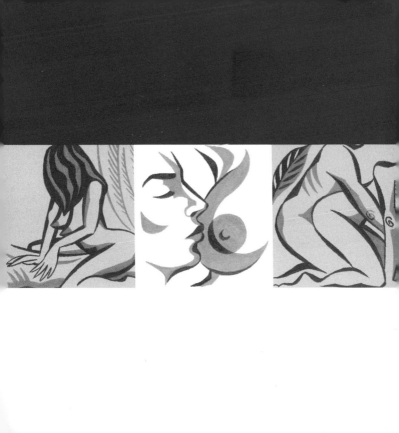

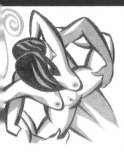 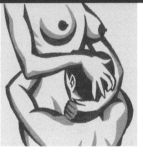 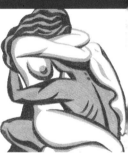

1 SEX AND SPIRITUALITY

Sexuality is the most powerful creative force we possess, as well as being a source of intense physical pleasure and emotional joy.

But sex can also be a path toward spiritual awakening. When you journey along this ancient path, sexual pleasure becomes a gateway to divine bliss.

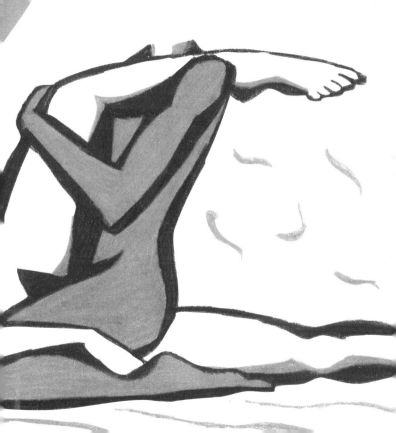

By bringing spirituality into the bedroom, you can use the passion and power of erotic energy to explore the connection between body, mind, and spirit.

Sex then evolves into a sacrament and a tool for transformation.

For when you discover the truly sacred nature of sex, you gain not only fulfilling passion and intimacy, but a deeper connection with yourself, your lover, and the divine spirit itself.

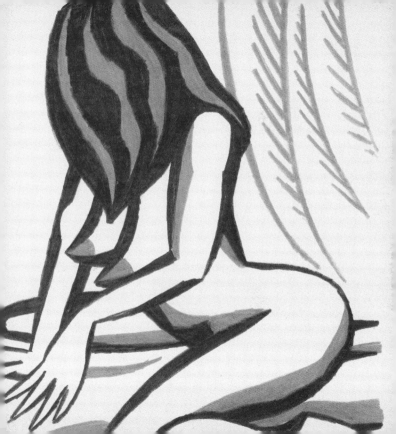

By transcending the purely physical and transforming sexual energy into spiritual energy, you connect with the source of everything.

Engaging in sacred sex allows you to move beyond the physical realm, to work with the core male and female energies within you. Whether you call them god and goddess, yin and yang, or dark and light, these forces can be integrated and harmonized through sexual intimacy.

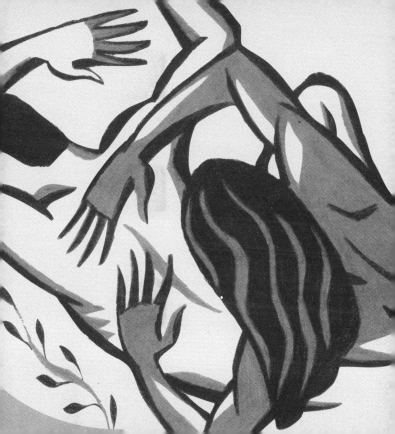

In orgasm we glimpse eternity—a sense of something greater than ourselves and earthly pleasures—and experience a timelessness and oneness with the universe.

By integrating spirituality with sexuality, we can turn that glimpse into a longer-lasting sense of awakening that extends far beyond the bedroom.

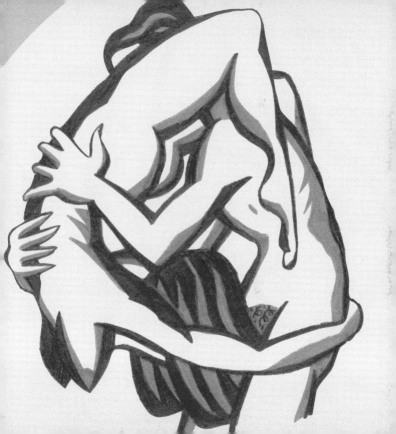

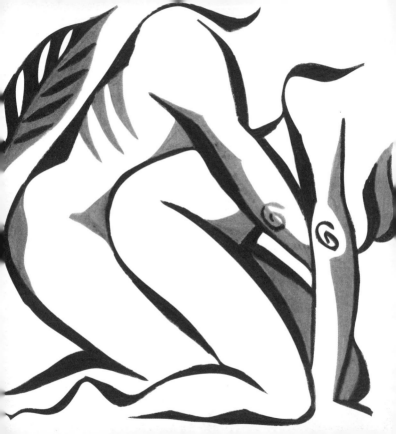

This book presents ideas from two ancient paths—Tantra and Taoism—which reveal that sexuality and spirituality are not only compatible, they are complementary.

Both spiritual traditions show that sex is not an obstacle to spiritual progress, but a stepping stone to help us along the path.

Tantra is a radical path that embraces direct life-experience as a liberating force, and uses desire, passion, and ecstasy as tools of enlightenment.

Tantrics teach that the everyday can be transformed into the divine if we approach all activities, including lovemaking, as an act of worship.

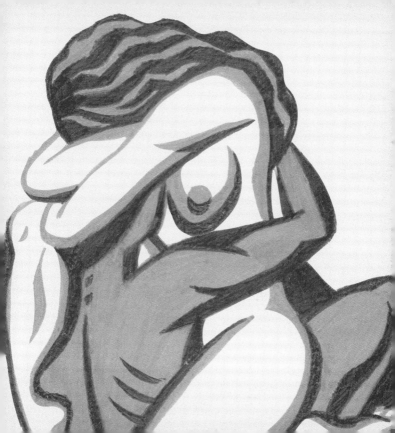

ONE MEANING OF TANTRA IS "EXPANSION": IT CELEBRATES THE WIDENING OF HORIZONS AND THE HEIGHTENING OF CONSCIOUSNESS THROUGH IMMERSION IN THE SENSUAL EXPERIENCE OF LIFE.

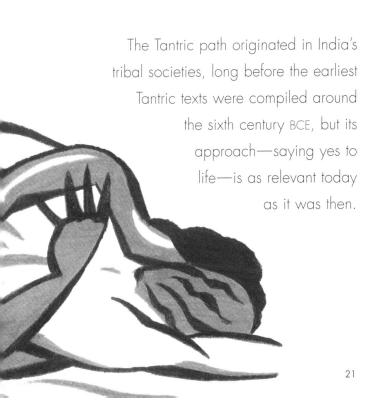

The Tantric path originated in India's
tribal societies, long before the earliest
Tantric texts were compiled around
the sixth century BCE, but its
approach—saying yes to
life—is as relevant today
as it was then.

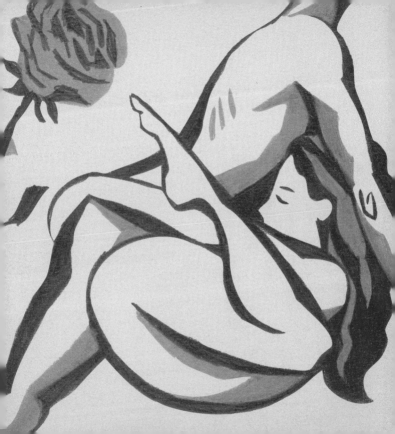

One of the founding fathers of Tantra was a learned monk, Saraha. One day he came across a woman arrow-maker in the marketplace, intent upon her work. She told him, "The Buddha's meaning can be known through symbols and actions, not through words and books."

Recognizing her as an enlightened presence, Saraha threw off his monastic vows and became her spiritual companion. He celebrated his new, humble lifestyle as the perfect context for spiritual practice and, on the day he and his arrow-maker lover were united, declared joyously, "Today I have become a true monk!"

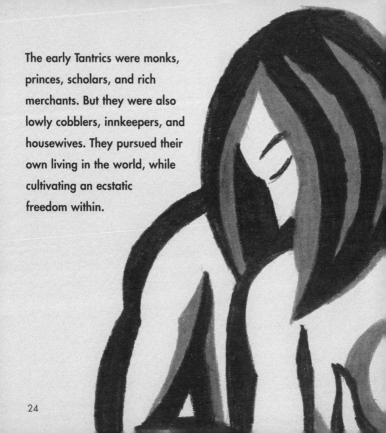

The early Tantrics were monks, princes, scholars, and rich merchants. But they were also lowly cobblers, innkeepers, and housewives. They pursued their own living in the world, while cultivating an ecstatic freedom within.

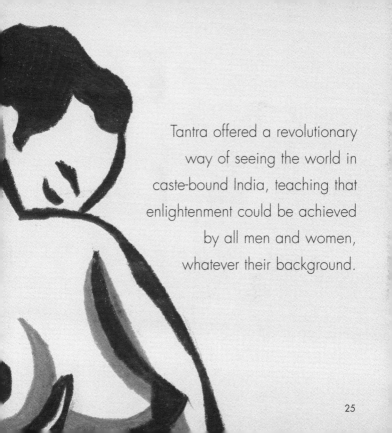

Tantra offered a revolutionary way of seeing the world in caste-bound India, teaching that enlightenment could be achieved by all men and women, whatever their background.

Through Tantra we
enter the realm of
the goddess.

Tantra teaches that the creative force behind all existence is female, in the form of the goddess Shakti, and that all women are honored as embodiments of the divine.

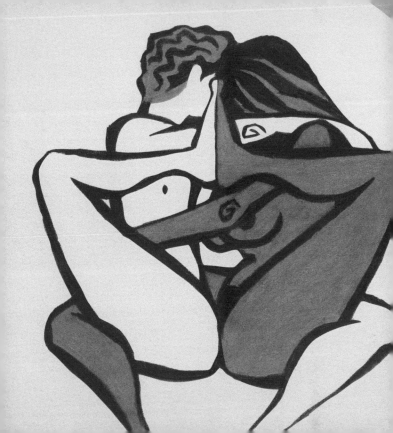

One should honor women.

Women are heaven,
women are truth,

Women are the supreme
fire of transformation.

Women are Buddha,
women are religious community,

Women are the
perfection of wisdom.

Candamaharosana Tantra

IN TANTRIC MYTHOLOGY, WHEN THE
GODDESS SHAKTI UNITFS WITH HER GOD,
SHIVA, THE ENTIRE WORLD IS CREATED IN
A SEXUAL DANCE OF BLISS.

AND WHEN WE SURRENDER FULLY TO EACH
OTHER IN LOVEMAKING, WE CONNECT WITH
THE SOURCE OF THE UNIVERSE.

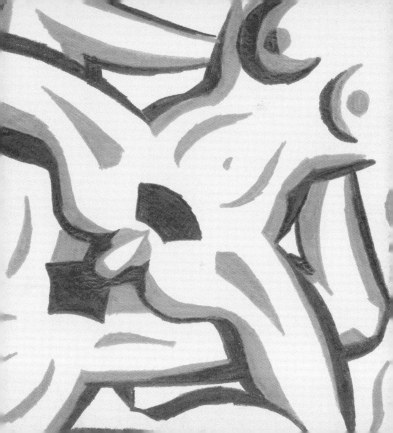

Tantric couples honor each other as goddess and god—the divine female and male principles—and use lovemaking as a way to channel and transform sexual energy into bliss, thereby liberating the soul.

For in the eyes of Tantra, we are all divine.

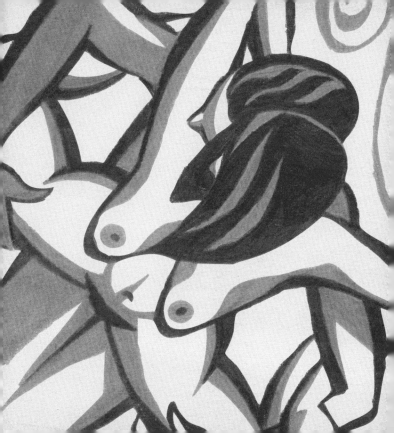

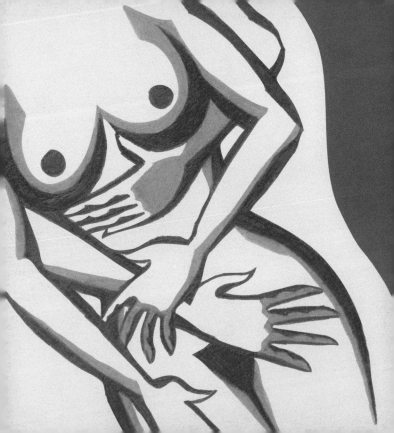

The Taoists of ancient China also saw lovemaking as part of the great eternal cosmic dance of two complementary energies in the universe—named yin and yang in this tradition.

They taught that sex is part of the natural order of life, and that lovemaking offers a way of bringing the opposite forces of yin and yang into harmony.

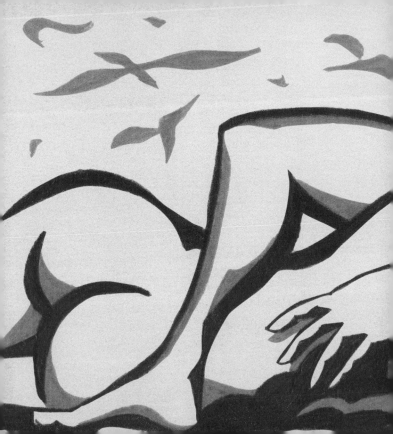

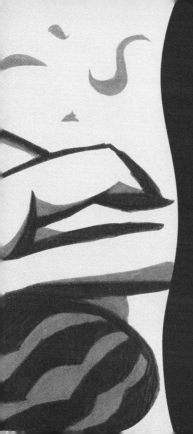

The ancient men and women of
the Tao were highly practical.
They looked at all the vital
elements of life—diet, exercise,
mankind's relationship with the
natural world—and sought to
find simple truths and ways of
behaving that allow each of us
to experience health, harmony,
and happiness.

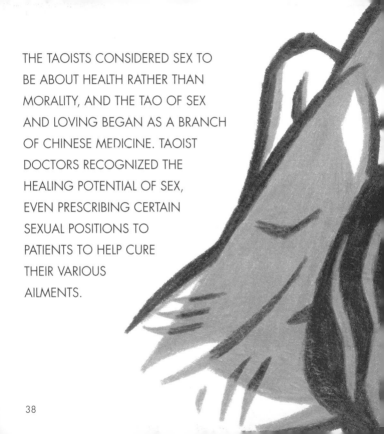

THE TAOISTS CONSIDERED SEX TO
BE ABOUT HEALTH RATHER THAN
MORALITY, AND THE TAO OF SEX
AND LOVING BEGAN AS A BRANCH
OF CHINESE MEDICINE. TAOIST
DOCTORS RECOGNIZED THE
HEALING POTENTIAL OF SEX,
EVEN PRESCRIBING CERTAIN
SEXUAL POSITIONS TO
PATIENTS TO HELP CURE
THEIR VARIOUS
AILMENTS.

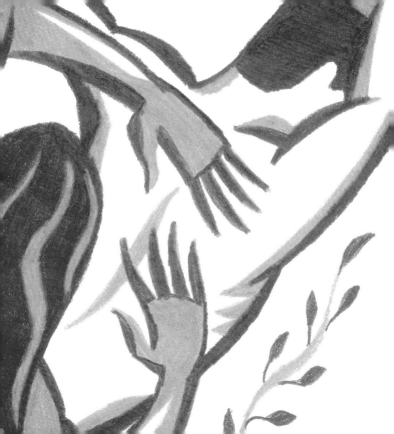

...no medicine or food
or spiritual salvation
can prolong a man's life
if he neither understands
nor practices the Tao
of Loving.

P'eng Tsu

For Taoists, healthy cultivatio

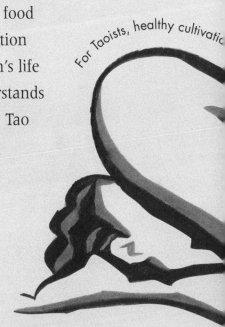

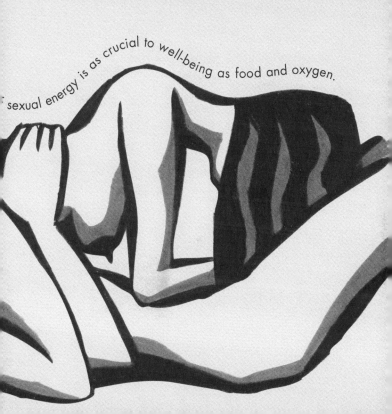

sexual energy is as crucial to well-being as food and oxygen.

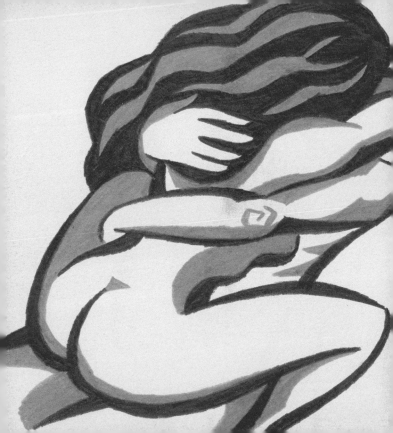

From earliest times, the Tao offered advice to help men and women nurture their sexual relationships in the most fulfilling way possible.

The Tao of loving understands that couples may have different sexual desires and rhythms, and teaches ways to harmonize those differences to create a profoundly satisfying and intimate love life.

TAOIST SEXUAL WISDOM OFFERS A HOLISTIC
APPROACH TO SEX, FAR REMOVED FROM THE
SEPARATION OF BODY, MIND, AND SPIRIT IN
THE WEST TODAY.

TAOISM TEACHES THAT SEXUAL ENERGY CAN BE
USED TO CULTIVATE EVERY OTHER ASPECT OF LIFE,
INCLUDING PHYSICAL HEALTH, EMOTIONAL
INTIMACY, AND SPIRITUAL GROWTH.

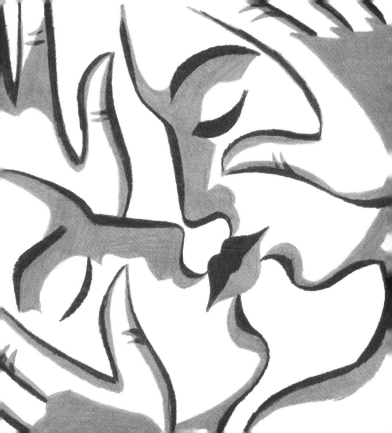

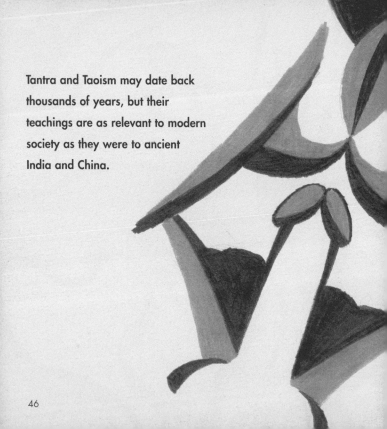

Tantra and Taoism may date back thousands of years, but their teachings are as relevant to modern society as they were to ancient India and China.

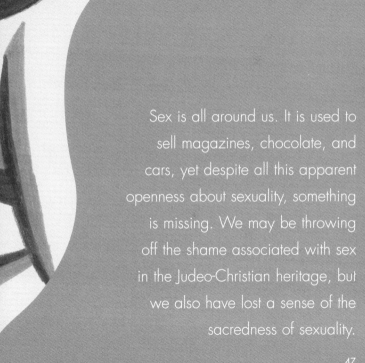

Sex is all around us. It is used to sell magazines, chocolate, and cars, yet despite all this apparent openness about sexuality, something is missing. We may be throwing off the shame associated with sex in the Judeo-Christian heritage, but we also have lost a sense of the sacredness of sexuality.

The link between our spirituality and sex lives is something the Tantric and Taoist masters understood well, and it is a link that many lovers today are struggling to rediscover.

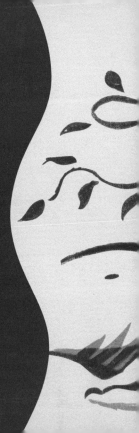

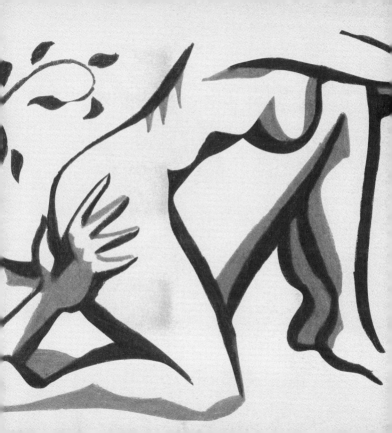

Spiritual Sex is a first step on the path to reintegrating your sexuality and spirituality.

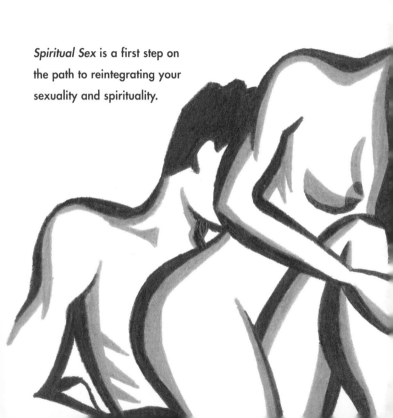

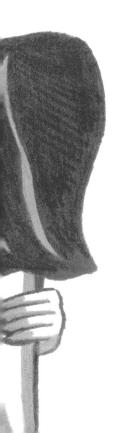

Here, words of sexual wisdom from traditional Tantric and Taoist works, as well as inspiration and advice from contemporary masters, sit alongside practical exercises and techniques to enhance your sex life.

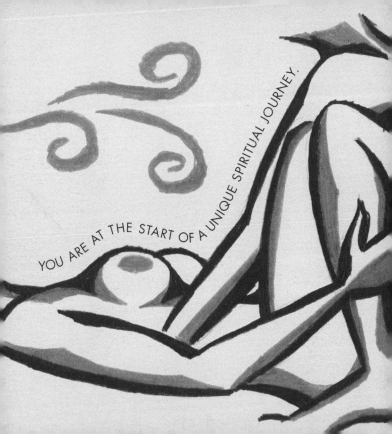

YOU ARE AT THE START OF A UNIQUE SPIRITUAL JOURNEY.

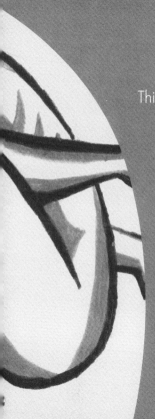

This book presents ideas to inspire you along the way. Some are simple; others may appear unusual or challenging. Follow your heart and your instinct: explore ideas where they appeal, make them your own, ask "what if?", and see what happens…

By practice, even without understanding, it will be made plain; your body will understand it long before your mind puts words to it. No amount of understanding without practice will work. It is not necessary that knowledge precedes experience. Performance will produce knowledge.

Shiva Sutra

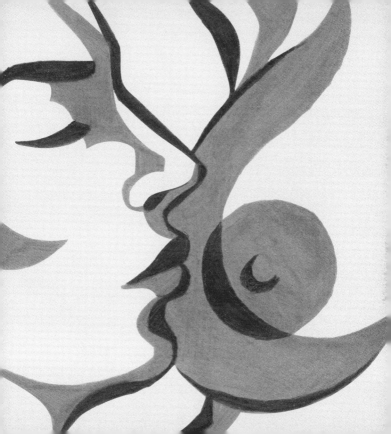

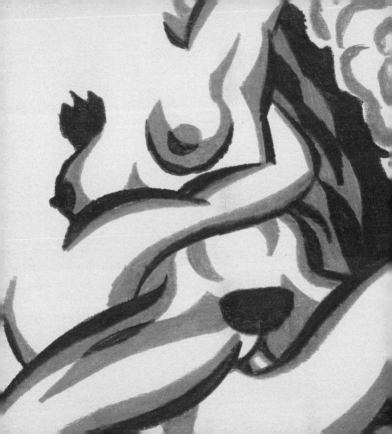

Spiritual sex is a path open to all—young or old, male or female, gay or straight. It requires no special vows, just an open mind and heart, and a willingness to embrace love and life to the full.

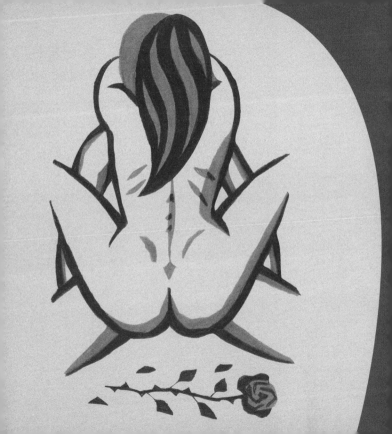

The only transformer
and alchemist

That turns everything
into gold is love.

Anais Nin

Making love with purpose and consciousness transforms sexual relationships; and, more than this, it reconnects us with our spiritual origins.

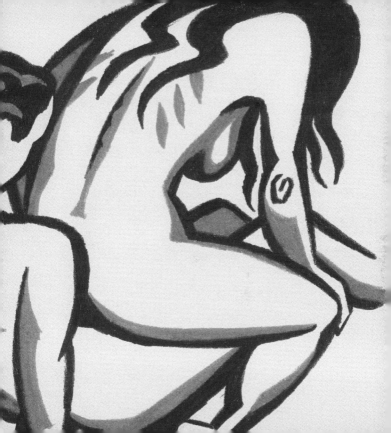

Spiritual sex is simply the start of the journey. Learning to feel the energy of creation within yourself and your partner during lovemaking offers an insight into the interconnectedness of all things. This is a gift that will stay with you, and permeate every part of your life.

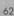

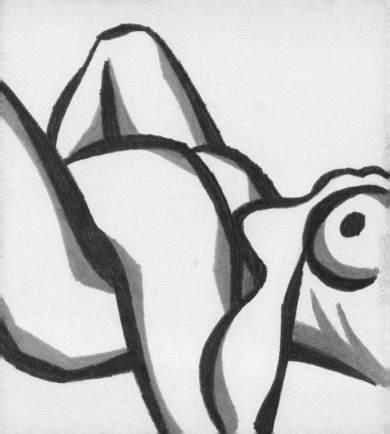

Love, enjoyed by the ignorant,
Becomes bondage.

That very same love,
Tasted by one with understanding,
Brings liberation.

Enjoy all the pleasures of love fearlessly,
For the sake of liberation.

Cittavisuddhoprakarana

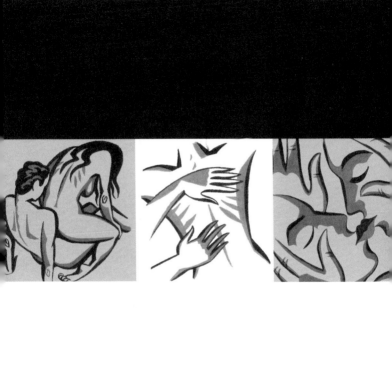

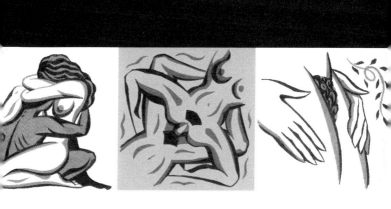

2 WEBS OF ENERGY

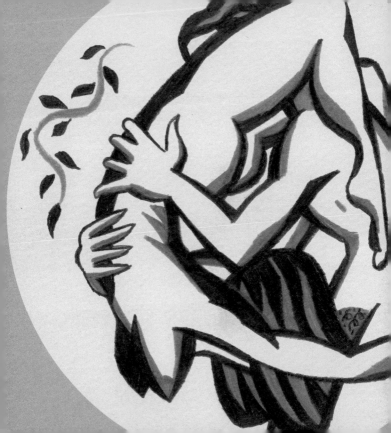

He who realizes the truth of the body can then come to know the truth of the universe.

Rat Nas Tantra

There is more to the body than its outward physical form. At its core is energy. Although this energy cannot easily be seen, it is the source of everything.

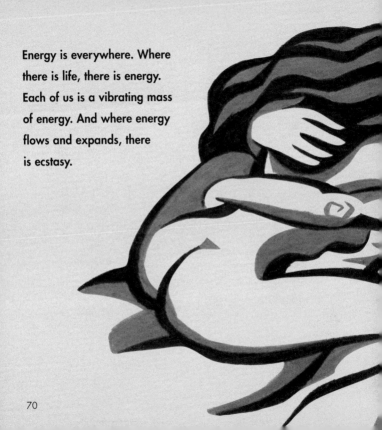

Energy is everywhere. Where
there is life, there is energy.
Each of us is a vibrating mass
of energy. And where energy
flows and expands, there
is ecstasy.

...Modern science has shown us that what we once took to be the material world is, when seen from another perspective, in fact a manifestation of pure energy. Our bodies depend upon having a source of energy (food) to function. We are bombarded with energy from the Sun and from other sources in our environment. As earthly creatures, we are energetic beings. And nowhere is this shown most than in our sexual lives.

Walt Whitman

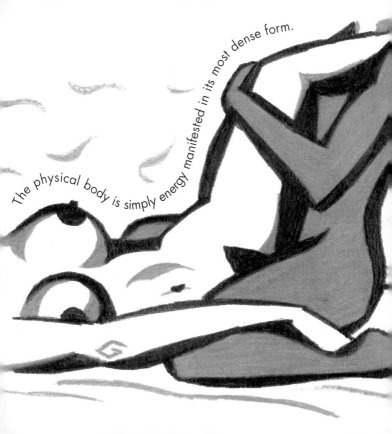

The physical body is simply energy manifested in its most dense form.

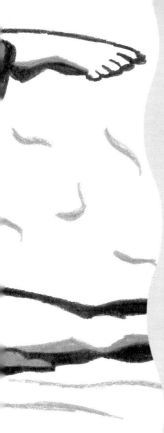

But energy moves in subtle ways, too. Within the body are sited powerful energy centers, known as chakras in the Indian Vedic system. A network of 14 invisible channels, called meridians in Traditional Chinese Medicine, carries energy to every part of the body. The chakras and meridians form the body's energy web. This subtle, or energy, body surrounds and permeates the physical body, drawing on the vital life-force around us and within us to nourish body, mind, and soul.

The ancient Tantrics and Taoists envisaged an invisible energy flowing through the universe, an essential life-force.

They called it prana in India, chi in China.

This is the vital energy and animating force of all things— humans, animals, nature, even the air we breathe.

It binds together the physical and subtle bodies, nourishing, replenishing, and attuning them, bringing mankind into harmony and balance with the universe.

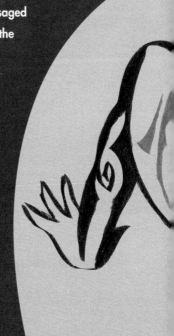

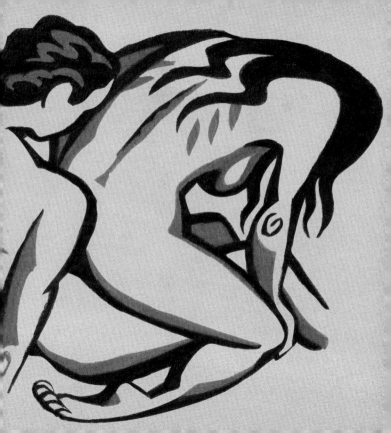

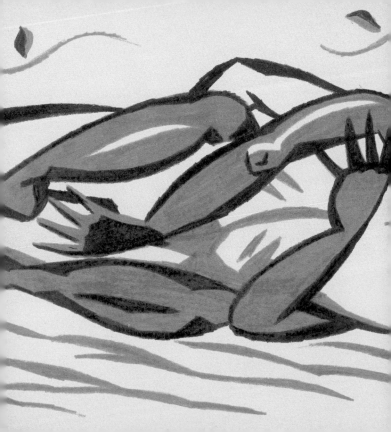

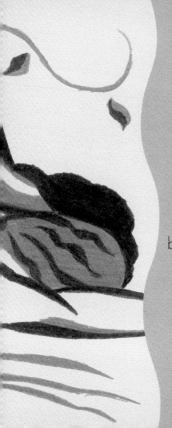

WHEN WE HAVE SEX,
TWO PHYSICAL BODIES
MEET AND UNITE,
BUT SIMULTANEOUSLY,
TWO ENERGETIC BODIES
DO THE SAME.

Being aware of your energy
body during lovemaking, and
working creatively with it,
allows you to transform your
physical experiences into
spiritual bliss.

77

The Subtle Body
connects this world with the next.
There is no single object or
doctrine as important and lasting
as the Subtle Body, which provides
a constant doorway to Liberation.

Kaula Tantra

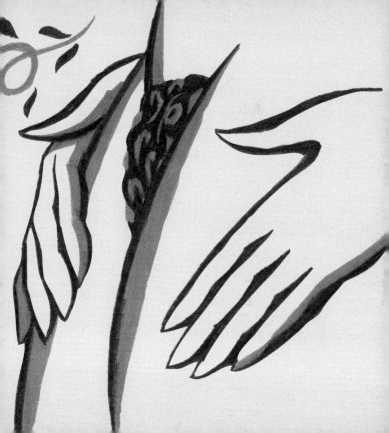

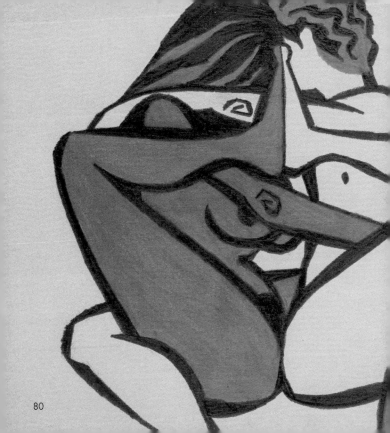

On an energy level, sex is a dance of opposites shared by lovers. The ultimate is to achieve harmony and beauty in this dance of the male and female principles, of yin and yang. This comes when both partners tune in to the dynamic balance of sexual play, and consciously share and circulate energies during lovemaking.

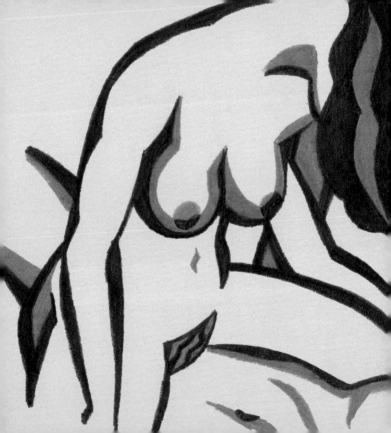

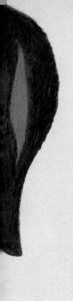

For thousands of years, a symbolic map of the body's energy web has been used to help people visualize and work with it more effectively.

IT IS KNOWN AS THE CHAKRA SYSTEM.

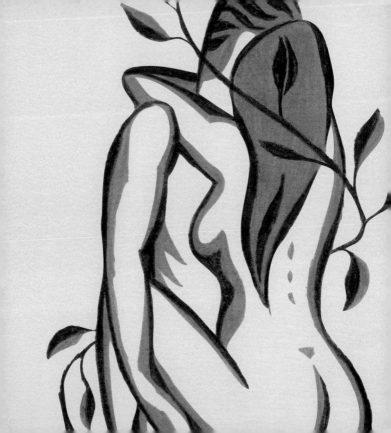

Chakras are energy centers situated on an invisible energy channel that runs alongside the spine. Each chakra is pictured as a spinning wheel of energy that draws in prana (life-force) from the energy flowing around us, and propels it upward to the chakra sited at the crown of the head—the gateway for self-realization.

CHAKRAS ARE JUNCTIONS FOR THE DYNAMIC INTERPLAY OF ENERGY AND CONSCIOUSNESS.

In Tantric thought, seven main chakras connect the physical body to the subtle body. Each corresponds to one aspect of physical nature, emotional being, and spiritual understanding. Each also has an associated element, color, and mantra (sacred sound).

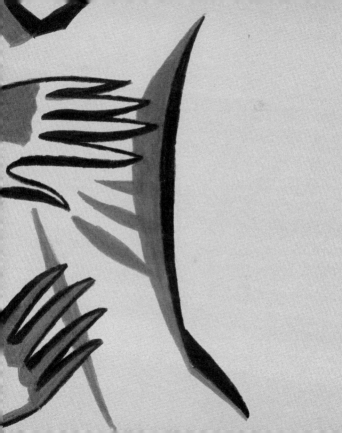

Root chakra

COLOR: red
ELEMENT: earth
MANTRA: lam

The first chakra is located at the base of the spine and is the home of sleeping kundalini energy, which is considered to be the creative force of the cosmos in the Hindu tradition. The root chakra governs instincts, and from here we experience a connection with the earth, and a sense of grounding and individuality.

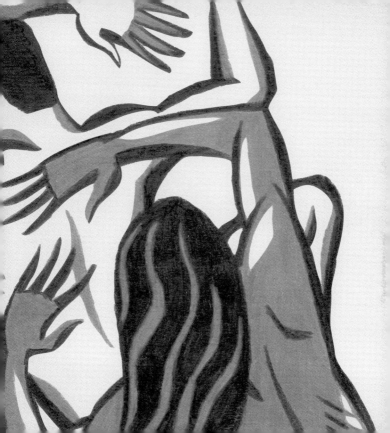

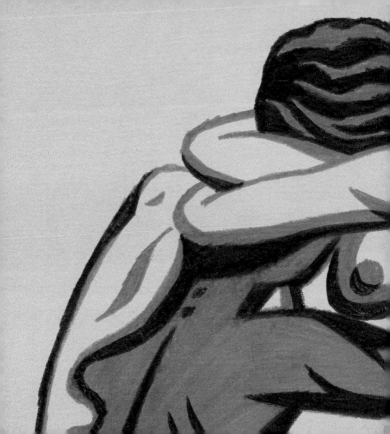

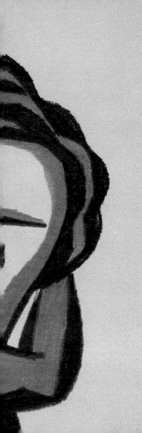

Sacral chakra

COLOR: orange
ELEMENT: water
MANTRA: vam

Located in the lower abdomen, the sacral or pelvic chakra is the watery source of pleasure, desire, and sexuality, and connects us with our emotions.

Solar/naval chakra

COLOR: yellow

ELEMENT: fire

MANTRA: ram

The fiery solar chakra is the home of personal power, trust, and respect. It gives a sense of "who I am," and transforms the earth and water energies of the first two chakras into action and power.

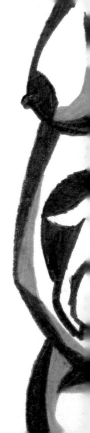

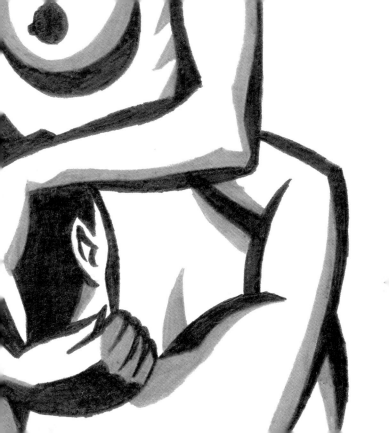

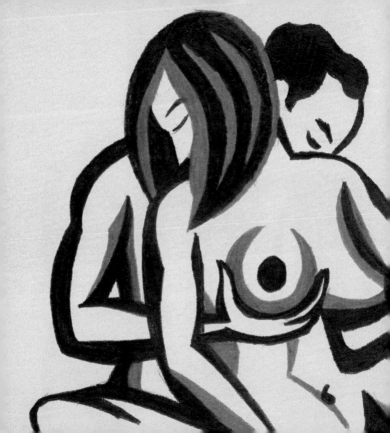

Heart chakra

COLOR: green
ELEMENT: air
MANTRA: yam

Located in the center of the chest, this chakra forms the bridge between body and consciousness. It is the focus for love, and corresponds to compassion and the ability to surrender. It governs the emotional, mystical, and unpredictable. The heart chakra frees energy to move upward, into the realms of bliss.

Throat chakra

COLOR: blue

ELEMENT: ether or space

MANTRA: ham

Communication and creativity
are associated with the throat
chakra, as well as inhalation,
exhalation, and balance.
Here, energy is expressed
and communicated to others.

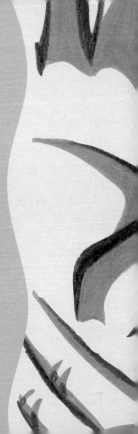

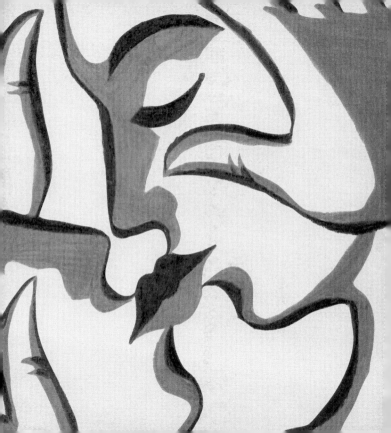

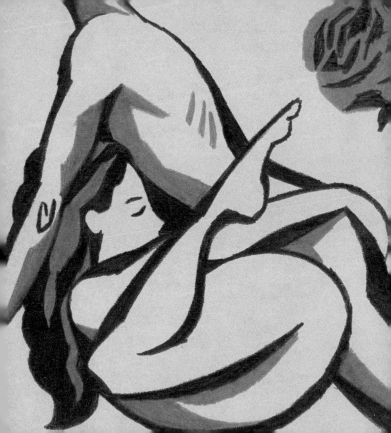

Third-eye chakra

COLOR: indigo
ELEMENT: light
MANTRA: om

The third eye, in the center of the forehead, represents perception, clairvoyance, and intellect. From here, imagination and intuition determine how we see the world around us—it is the site of sudden insights.

Crown chakra

The crown chakra, at the top of the head, is the home of the divine, the site of union and wisdom. Its energies are cool and mystical, and it has no associated element or mantra. It is the seat of the soul.

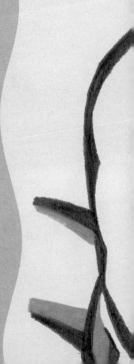

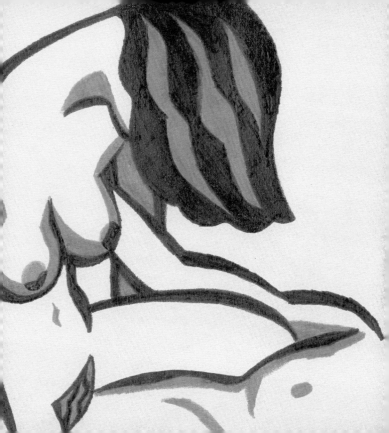

Look at these worlds spinning out of nothingness.

That is your power.

Rumi

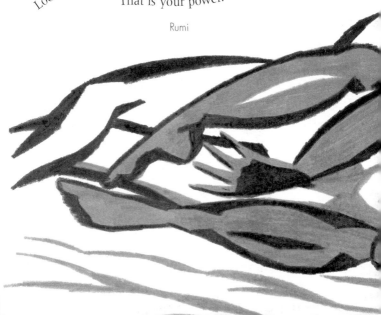

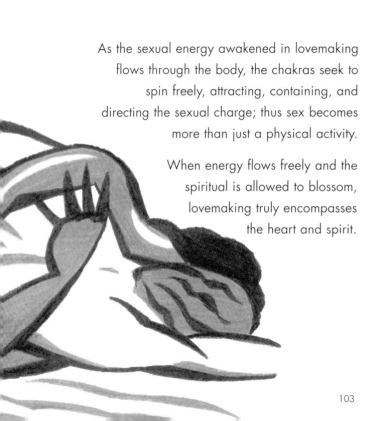

As the sexual energy awakened in lovemaking flows through the body, the chakras seek to spin freely, attracting, containing, and directing the sexual charge; thus sex becomes more than just a physical activity.

When energy flows freely and the spiritual is allowed to blossom, lovemaking truly encompasses the heart and spirit.

PRACTICE THIS SIMPLE EXERCISE TO
ATTUNE YOU TO YOUR CHAKRAS:
VISUALIZE EACH CHAKRA IN TURN AS A
LOTUS FLOWER SLOWLY UNFOLDING.

Start with the root chakra, imagining it
unfold, then move up the body, focusing
your awareness on each energy center
in turn. Feel the energy spinning inside
each chakra, and see its color glowing
brighter. Try intoning each chakra's
mantra as you exhale, visualizing your
breath filling the chakra with color and
energy when you inhale.

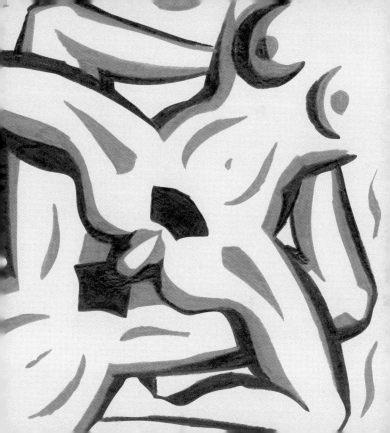

After opening your chakras, try this easy exercise for closing them again. Visualize each chakra as a stained-glass window of the appropriate color.

Imagine drawing energy down from your crown chakra, and feel it flow over each chakra in turn, closing them off like a white shutter coming down over the window. You might need to draw on more energy from the crown as you move down the body.

Leave the root and crown chakras open to absorb energy.

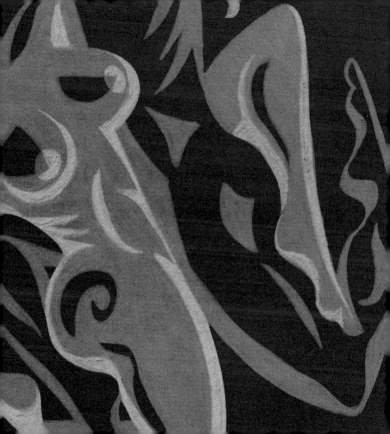

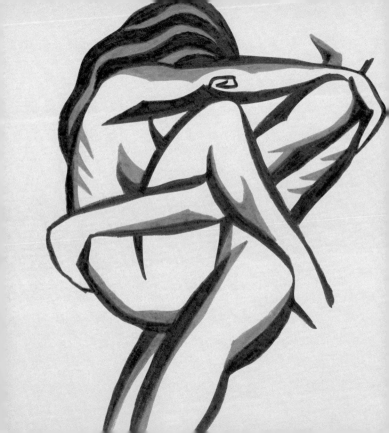

When we make love, a powerful, creative energy is able to journey up the path linking the chakras, connecting energy focused in the body with consciousness.

Called kundalini, this energy is our powerhouse of life-force, and the source of the creative process.

Visualized as a coiled serpent of potential energy, this force sleeps at the base of the spine, waiting to be awakened and drawn upward to create an intense state of spiritual ecstasy.

KUNDALINI CAN BE AWAKENED
THROUGH DANCE, PHYSICAL
ACTIVITY SUCH AS YOGA, OR EVEN
SOUND. BUT IT IS THROUGH
TRANSCENDENTAL LOVEMAKING
THAT THE SERPENT GODDESS
CREATES HER MOST MAGICAL
ALCHEMY, TRANSFORMING SIMPLE
PHYSICAL UNION INTO MYSTICAL
ONENESS WITH THE UNIVERSE.

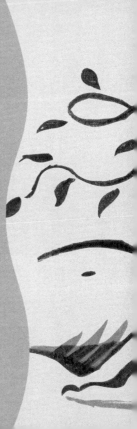

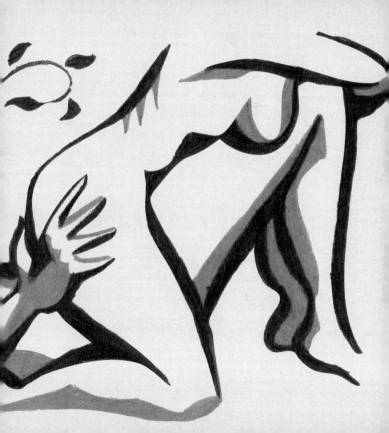

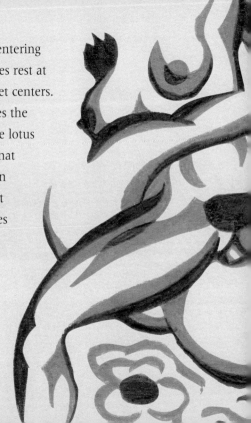

The inner woman, entering the 'royal road,' takes rest at intervals in the secret centers. Finally She embraces the Supreme Lord in the lotus of the head. From that union there flows an exquisite nectar that floods and permeates the body; then the Ineffable Bliss is experienced.

Anandagiri

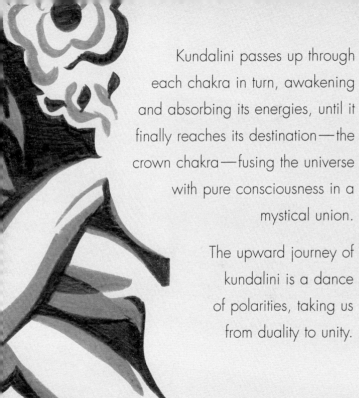

Kundalini passes up through each chakra in turn, awakening and absorbing its energies, until it finally reaches its destination—the crown chakra—fusing the universe with pure consciousness in a mystical union.

The upward journey of kundalini is a dance of polarities, taking us from duality to unity.

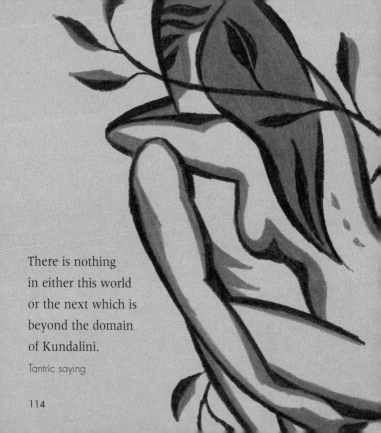

There is nothing
in either this world
or the next which is
beyond the domain
of Kundalini.

Tantric saying

KUNDALINI IS THE GODDESS OF ENERGY
WITHIN BOTH MEN AND WOMEN.

SHE IS THE SOURCE OF SEXUALITY, CREATIVITY,
FERTILITY, AND TRANSFORMATION.

THROUGH KUNDALINI WE CAN CONNECT
WITH THE ENERGY OF THE COSMOS.

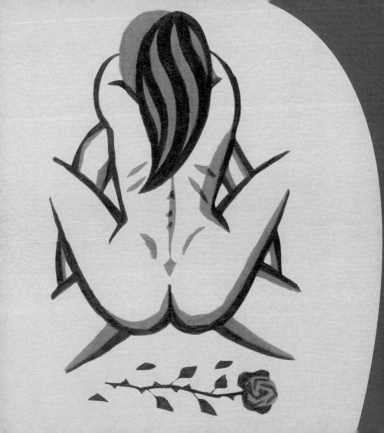

Bring awareness to your Kundalini powerhouse with a simple shaking exercise.

Stand with feet shoulder-width apart, knees soft, arms loose and eyes closed. Now take some deep breaths, in through the nose and out through the mouth.

Start to shake your pelvis and hips while keeping your knees soft and feet firm. Allow the shaking to move up through every part of your body. Keep breathing deeply and let your body tremble like a leaf in the wind.

Some rhythmic music helps!

Continue for as long as you feel comfortable, before lying down and enjoying the feeling of surging energy within.

When the sleeping goddess Kundalini is awakened through the grace of the teacher, then all the subtle lotuses and worldly bonds are readily pierced through and through. Let the wise person forcibly and firmly draw up the goddess Kundalini, for She is the giver of miraculous powers.

Shiva Samhita

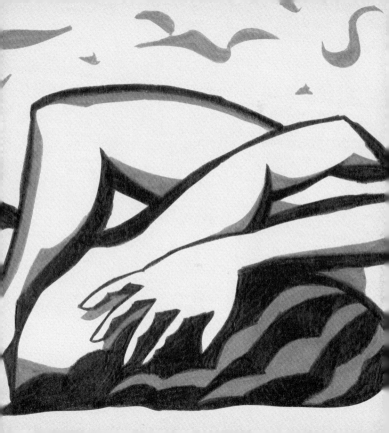

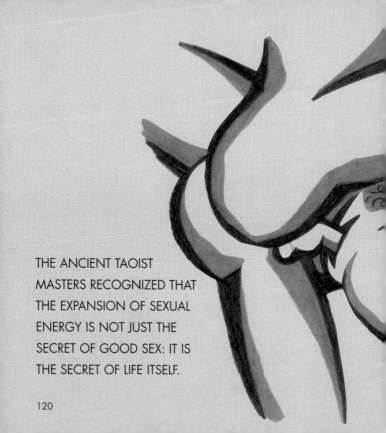

THE ANCIENT TAOIST
MASTERS RECOGNIZED THAT
THE EXPANSION OF SEXUAL
ENERGY IS NOT JUST THE
SECRET OF GOOD SEX: IT IS
THE SECRET OF LIFE ITSELF.

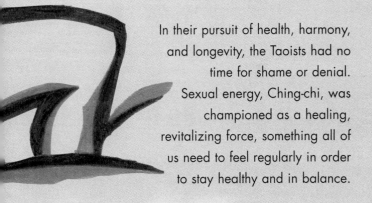

In their pursuit of health, harmony, and longevity, the Taoists had no time for shame or denial. Sexual energy, Ching-chi, was championed as a healing, revitalizing force, something all of us need to feel regularly in order to stay healthy and in balance.

The mind moves and the chi follows.

Taoist saying

Ching-chi is generated in the pelvic area. Directed by the mind, it can be drawn up the body and circulated through the natural circuits (meridians) in the body's energy web to provide a reservoir of powerful energy with which to nurture pleasure, health, and spiritual growth.

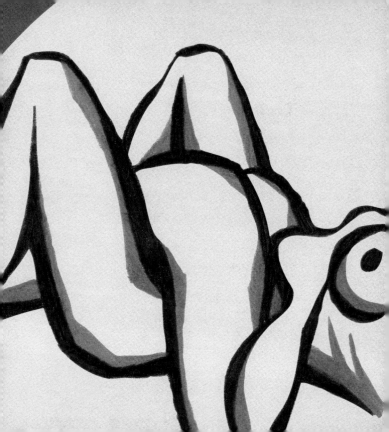

Your genitals and spine are like a water wheel that draws the energy up your spine and then pours it into your head to replenish your brain. From there it flows down like a waterfall into your abdomen, where it can be stored in a life-giving reservoir of energy. The Taoists knew there is nothing more powerful than water and nothing more powerful in our body than our sexual energy.

Mantak Chia

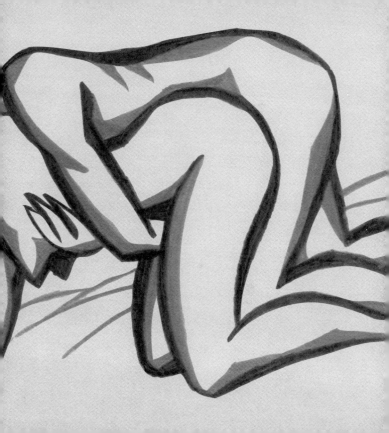

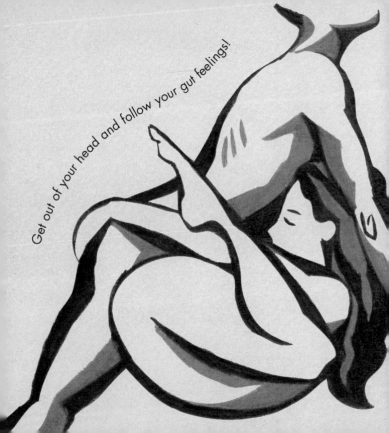

Get out of your head and follow your gut feelings!

There are reservoirs of energy in the brain, heart, and abdomen, but because we tend to expend most energy in the brain, many people get "stuck" in the head. The Taoists teach the importance of shifting the focus to the "second brain," the abdomen. Here, energy is stored and released most effectively, like a time-release capsule.

In becoming aware of the energy body, we start to understand how lovemaking connects us to energies deep within us. A spark of bliss unites the cosmic female and male principles—yin and yang—within us all, connecting us to the sacred source of all matter.

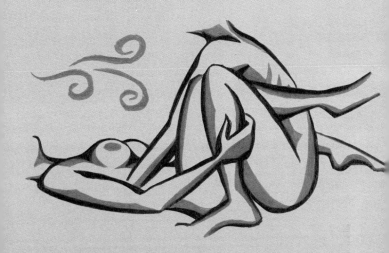

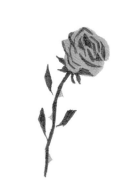

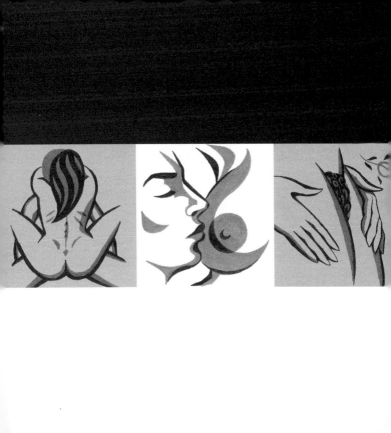

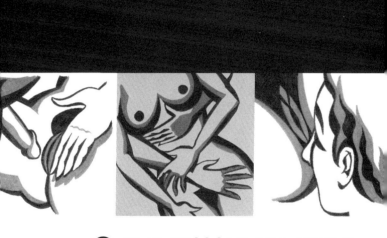

3 THE **FEMALE** PRINCIPLE

THROUGH SPIRITUAL SEX WE ENTER
THE REALM OF THE GODDESS.

In ancient Tantra and Taoism,
woman is recognized and
honored as the womb of
creation, the womb of all life,
and it is women who are the
keepers and transmitters of
sexual secrets. Independent,
enlightened women were among the
key founders of Tantra, and three of the
most important figures in the Taoist
teachings on sex are the Yellow Emperor's
triad of outspoken female initiators.

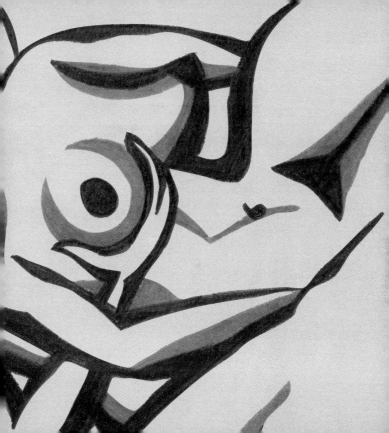

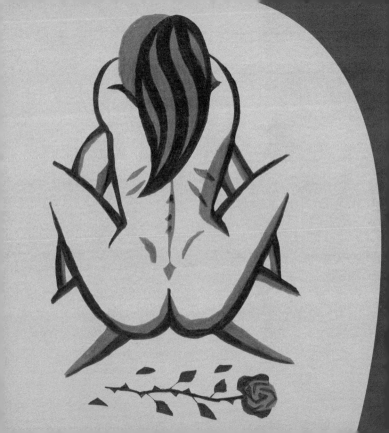

Woman is the creator of the universe.

The universe is her form;

Woman is the foundation of the world,

She is the true form of the body.

Whatever form she takes,

Whether the form of a man or a woman,

Is the superior form.

Saktisangama Tantra

Tantrics worship every woman as the
embodiment of the goddess Shakti, the
creative force behind existence.

Being pure energy, the goddess Shakti takes on the form of various female deities, who represent the different qualities of her primal energy.

She might be the temptress Mohini, the divine seductress who initiated the act of love responsible for creation, Gauri, the deity representing purity and austerity, or Kali, the goddess of destruction. In her creative aspect she is Saraswati, the patron of the 64 arts one should cultivate in life, including the art of loving.

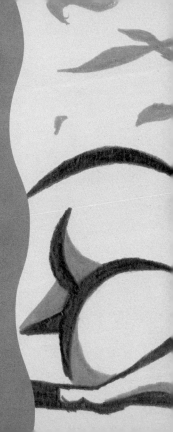

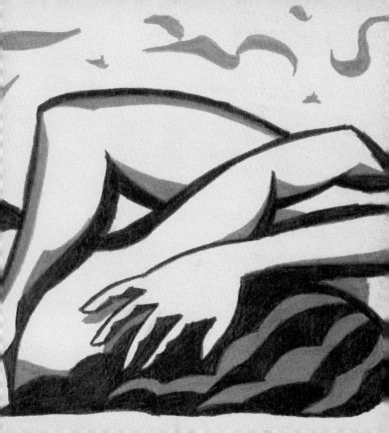

As the awe-inspiring and fearless Kali, the goddess represents the destructive phase of the eternal cycle of birth, death, and rebirth.

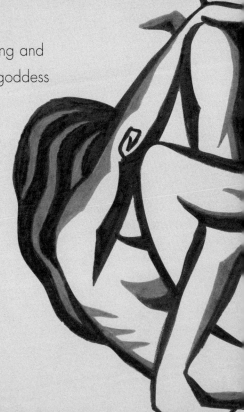

In this form she is the manifestation of the transcendental nature of womanhood, and can be found dancing on the corporeal body of her lover, the god Shiva.

Every woman has the goddess within her, and every time you awaken her you become fully in touch with your power as a woman.

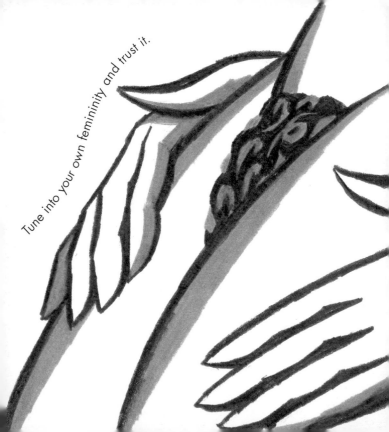

Tune into your own femininity and trust it.

The place to start is where you are right now. Nurture your goddess within by bringing beauty and sensuality into your everyday life. Be alive to the erotic possibilities all around you in art and in nature.

Feel the sun on your skin, hear the wind in your ears, appreciate the scent of flowers, the sound of sensual music. Feel your inner goddess and sexual energy awakening with the beauty of the world.

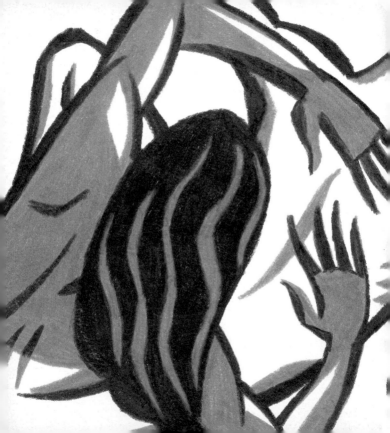

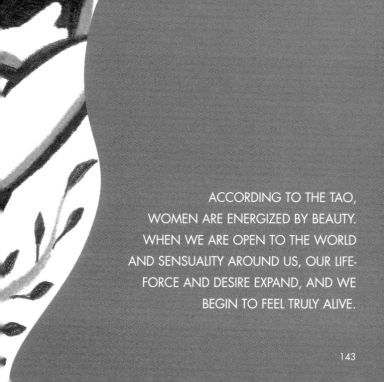

ACCORDING TO THE TAO,
WOMEN ARE ENERGIZED BY BEAUTY.
WHEN WE ARE OPEN TO THE WORLD
AND SENSUALITY AROUND US, OUR LIFE-
FORCE AND DESIRE EXPAND, AND WE
BEGIN TO FEEL TRULY ALIVE.

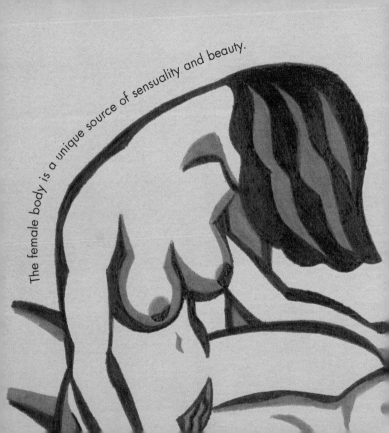

The female body is a unique source of sensuality and beauty.

How often do you look at your naked body with an uncritical and really appreciative gaze? Try it now—stand in front of a full-length mirror and celebrate the wonder that is your physical form. Turn off your critical gaze and recognize that you are perfect as you are and that all you need is within you.

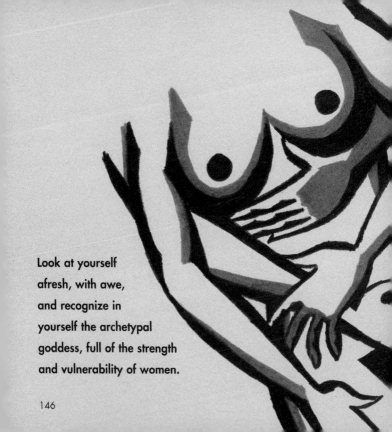

Look at yourself
afresh, with awe,
and recognize in
yourself the archetypal
goddess, full of the strength
and vulnerability of women.

146

Rejoice in your womanliness. Revel in your curves and softness, and relish your flesh. Run your hands over your body, feeling the weight of your breasts, the roundness of your belly, and the curve of your hips. Shake your buttocks, let your body move freely, and breathe love into every part of yourself.

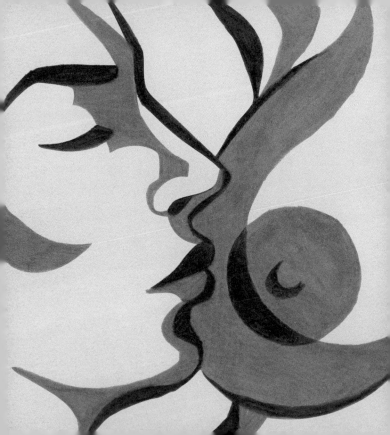

Feel the fine qualities of creativity permeating your breasts and assuming delicate configurations.

Osho

The breast meditation is a very powerful meditation for women, taught by the Indian teacher Osho.

Sit quietly, take a few deep breaths, and move your total consciousness to your breasts. Become one with them, forgetting the rest of your body. Relax and melt into them, and allow a sense of deep sweetness to envelop you, pulsating all around and within you.

Yoni is the Sanskrit word for the female sexual organs and means "sacred space." The "cosmic yoni" is an ancient sexual image, worshiped throughout history and various cultures as the source of life.

In Tantra, the yoni is worshiped as the sacred gateway to direct experience of the divine.

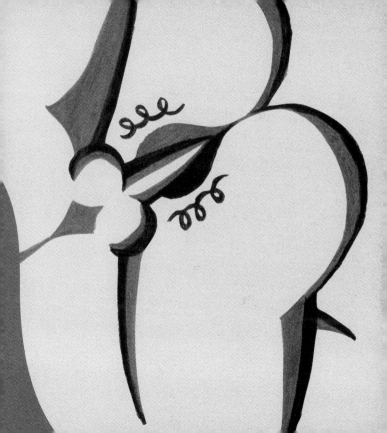

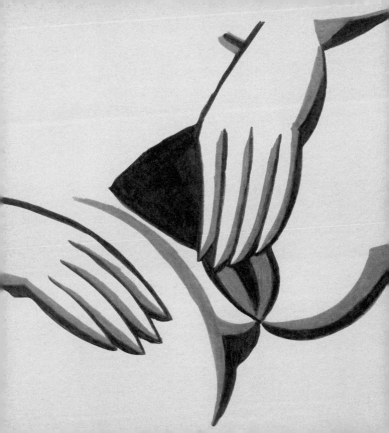

Take a mirror and really look at this sacred part of your body, the source of creation and pleasure. Explore this divine gateway with your gaze and touch; honor it as a temple of erotic love.

As you place your hands over your yoni, send warmth and love inward, and feel the powerful, mysterious energy emanating from within. Think about the memories stored up there, and use your loving gaze and touch as an honoring and, if necessary, healing process.

Masturbation, or self-pleasuring, is essential in Tantra as a means of self-knowing. It is not something shameful or dirty, but a voyage of self-discovery and exploration, the most natural way of loving yourself and enjoying your body to the full.

WHEN YOU HAVE EXPLORED AND REALLY KNOW YOUR BODY, YOU HOLD THE KEY TO SEXUAL ECSTASY.

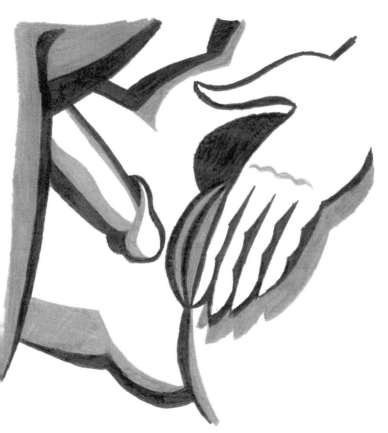

EXPERIENCE THE PLEASURE
OF SEDUCING YOURSELF,
THE LIBERATION OF BEING
BOTH ADORER AND ADORED.

Prepare a warm and inviting
space with candles and soft
music, as if you were awaiting
a lover. Take a warm bath, then start
to massage your skin with scented oils.
Use various strokes and explore how
different areas of skin respond to your
touch. Begin to arouse yourself, and feel
all inhibitions dissolve as the sensations
spread throughout your body.

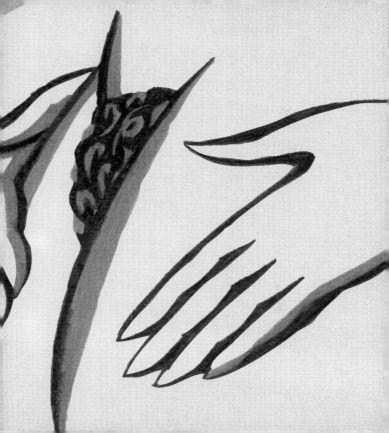

Use self-pleasuring to discover your own unique pattern of sexual arousal and to become fully aware of your orgasmic potential.

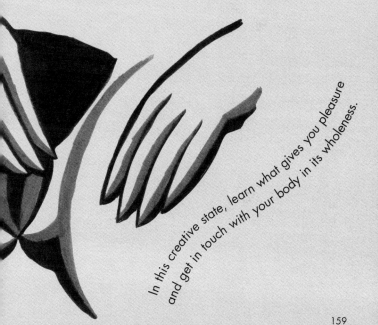

In this creative state, learn what gives you pleasure and get in touch with your body in its wholeness.

159

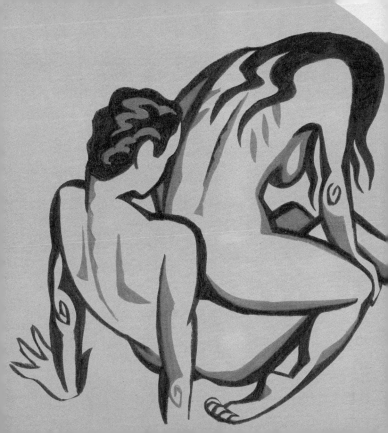

As you delight in the pleasures of your own flesh, you discover your own raw, earthy sexuality and instinctual sensuality.

From this comes sexual self-confidence; if you are not confident about what you need, how can you help someone else give you pleasure?

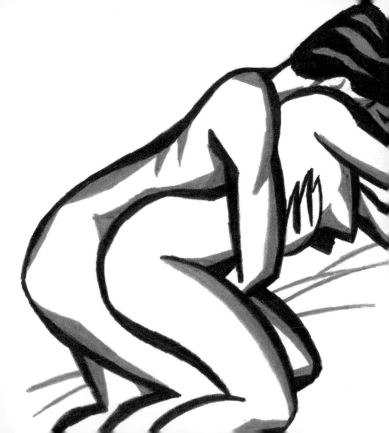

The ancient Tantric masters knew of a sacred spot inside the yoni long before Dr Grafenberg "discovered" the G-spot in the 1940s.

Deep inside and well hidden, it is a slightly more ridged, spongy area of tissue just under the pubic bone and behind the clitoris, which can be stroked and circled with the middle finger in a slightly curled position.

Once awakened, it is the source of profound pleasure and Shakti power. Tantrics even name it the "goddess spot" for its amazing power to bring women to peak states of arousal.

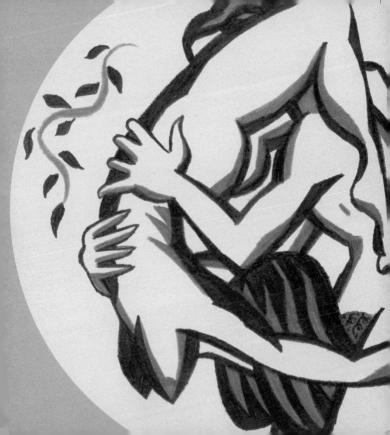

THE G-SPOT AND THE
CLITORIS ARE TWO CHARGED
SEXUAL POLES OF PLEASURE—
GATEWAYS TO DIVINE SEX.

When the goddess spot is awakened, a light, clear liquid may be released, which Tantrics call "divine love nectar" and Taoists know as "moon flower water".

The ancient texts recommend that men taste this nectar, worshiping their lover by drinking the most powerful yin essence from the yoni, the opening to life.

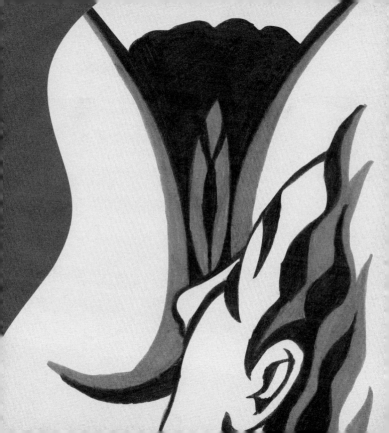

The eternal feminine draws us upward.

Goethe

The valley spirit never dies;
It is the woman, primal mother.
Her gateway is the root of
heaven and earth...

Lao Tsu

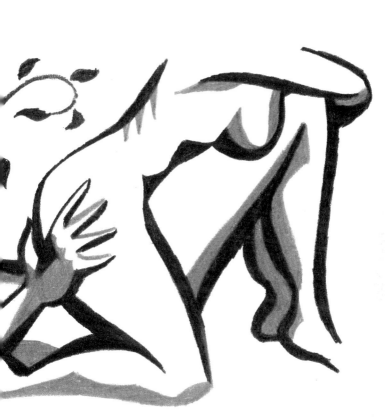

In Tantric lore, during menstruation a woman becomes a portal to other worlds.

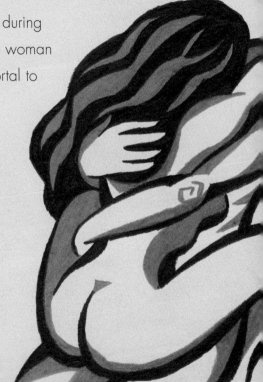

She is the embodiment of the goddess Kali, personifying transcendence and the renewing and regenerative power of female sexuality.

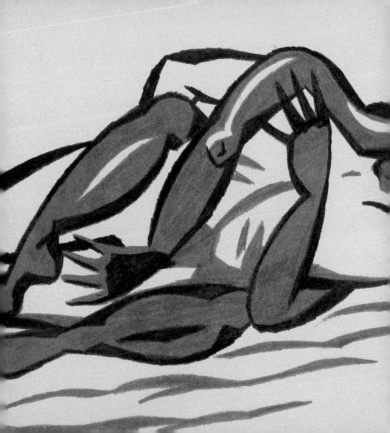

The Tantric adept should view a menstruating woman with reverence and awe. She is the living embodiment of Kali, the power of transcendence; her menstrual blood is the flowery essence of all womanhood, the very blood of life. Possessed of supernormal qualities, it is a potent rejuvenating and transforming force, purifying all poisons through its alchemical fire.

Kaula Tantra

Menstruation is a time of letting go,
cleansing, and renewal. Give yourself
space to reconnect with your body, with
your softness, and with your strength during
this potent phase of your natural cycle.

Let yourself be reborn each month.

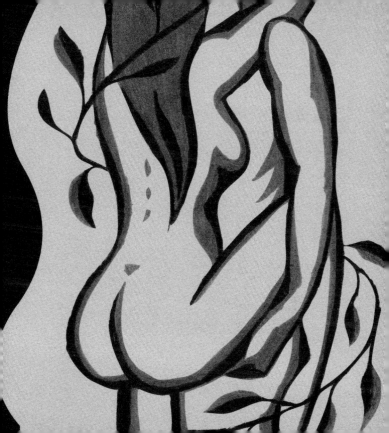

Look upon woman as a Goddess,
whose special energy she is,
and honor her in that state
of goddess.

Utara Tantra

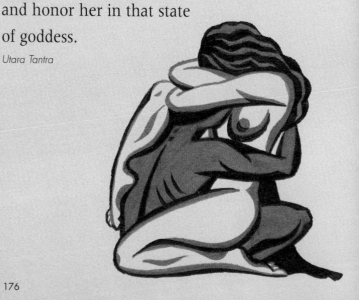

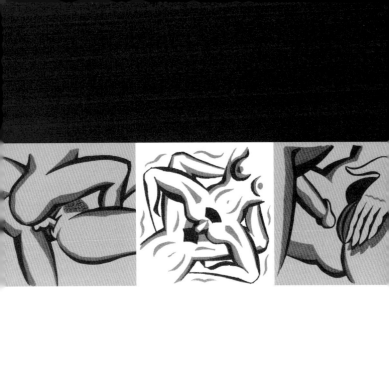

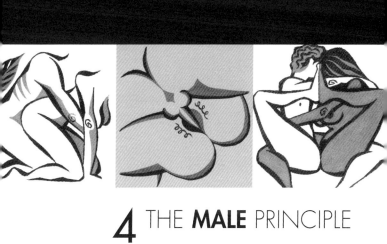

4 THE **MALE** PRINCIPLE

Yang energy is considered the primary force that binds the universe together.

In Taoist thought, the masculine energy of the cosmos is yang. This male vital energy is symbolized by fire and heaven. It is light and hard in quality, and dynamically active.

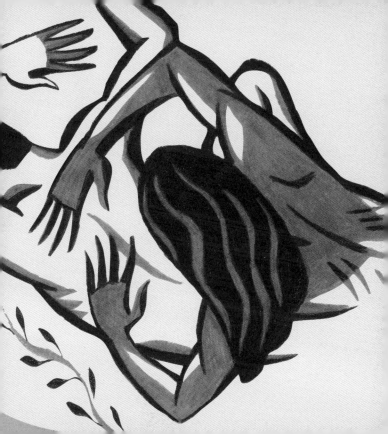

The subtle center situated at the base of the spine is a triangle of desire, knowledge, and action, which forms the womb at whose heart rises the phallus that is born of its own self, shining like a thousand suns.

Shiva Purana

JUST AS THE WOMAN'S YONI IS HONORED IN SACRED SEX, SO THE MAN'S PENIS IS REVERED AS A SYMBOL OF POWER AND CREATIVITY.

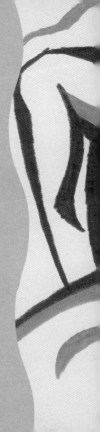

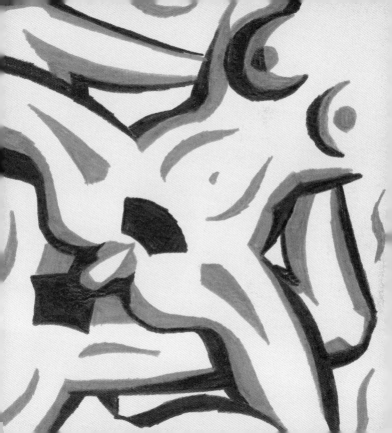

In Tantra, the penis
is called the lingam,
which has the
wonderful meaning
"wand of light." It is the
symbol of Shiva, the male
energy of consciousness.

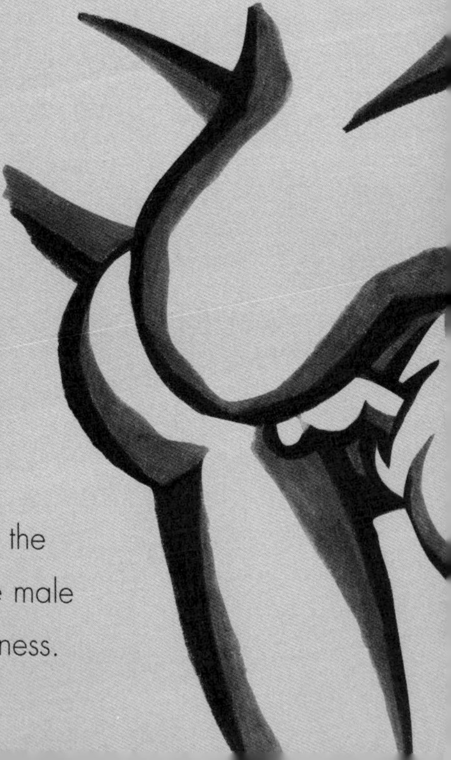

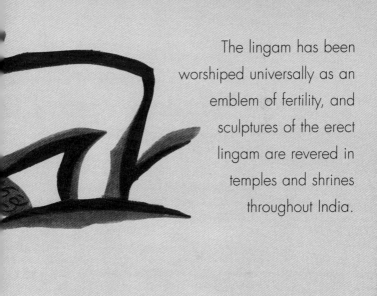

The lingam has been worshiped universally as an emblem of fertility, and sculptures of the erect lingam are revered in temples and shrines throughout India.

The whole universe was created from the seed that poured from the erect Lingam of Shiva during his lovemaking. All the gods worship that Lingam, the symbol of Lord Shiva, the Supreme Yogi.

Mahabharata

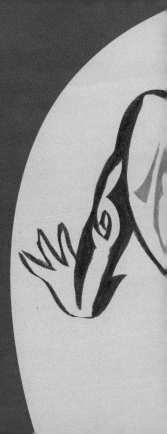

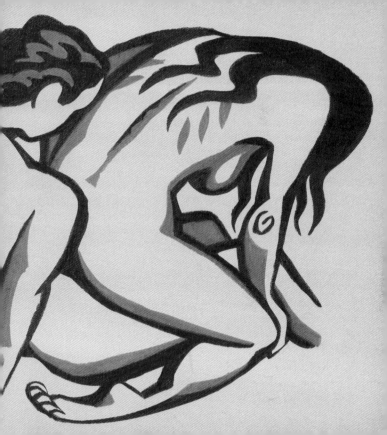

Being pure consciousness, Lord Shiva is transcendent and other-worldly. He needs the goddess Shakti to give him form, just as she needs him to give her consciousness. And so Shiva and Shakti act as complementary forces, requiring union with each other to achieve wholeness.

The coming together of Shakti and Shiva is the blissful union of energy and consciousness, and in Tantra, the entire physical and transcendental world is said to be generated by the sexual interplay of Shakti and Shiva.

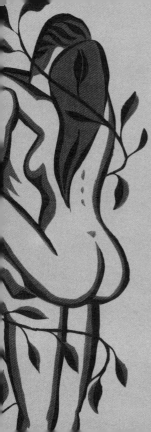

Behold the Shiva Lingam,
beautiful as molten gold,
firm as the Himalaya
Mountain, tender as a folded
leaf, life-giving like the
solar orb; behold the charm
of his sparkling jewels!

Linga Purana

Male power is rooted in the eternal cycle of birth, death, and rebirth as manifested in the male body. This cycle is embodied in the magical way the lingam moves from hard to soft and back again—it rises, swells, spurts, falls, and eventually rises again.

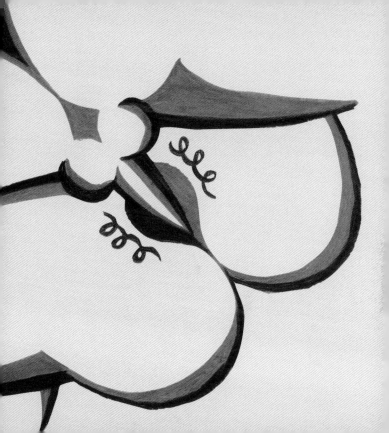

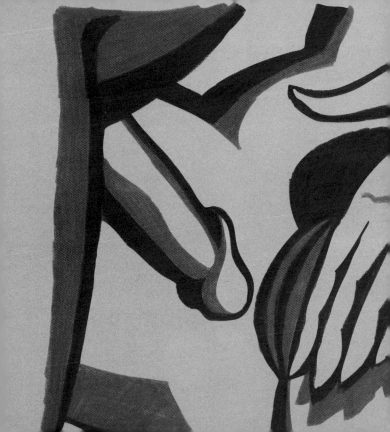

ACHIEVING THE MAGICAL BALANCE BETWEEN
HARDNESS AND SOFTNESS IS THE KEY
TO UNCOVERING YOUR FULL
POTENTIAL AS A MAN.

Men are socially conditioned from an
early age to hold back tears and
emotion, to develop only a "hard"
side and to bury softness. Yet, as
well as containing yang energy,
every man holds a store of
feminine yin energy within
that is vital for the eternal
dance of yin and yang.

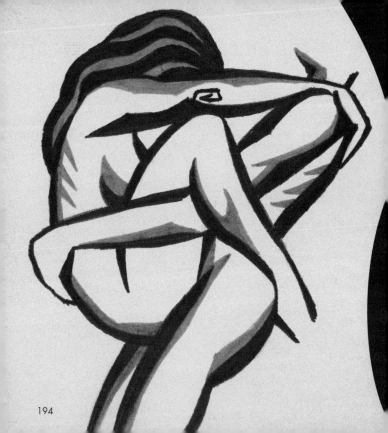

True male strength lies in getting in touch with the point of balance in the interplay of yin and yang. Try and embrace your vulnerability and sensitivity while opening up to the unique strength and power you embody as a man. In merging male and female aspects, you become fully alive.

A lingam meditation can help put you in touch with your inner power and vulnerability, and let you begin to heal past hurt.

Sitting comfortably, bring your awareness to the root of your lingam inside your body. Imagine it as an opening, perhaps filled with light or color. Steady your mind and focus on the sensations you experience and the energy you might feel stirring. Listen with respect to what this area of the body is trying to say to you, and acknowledge what you hear.

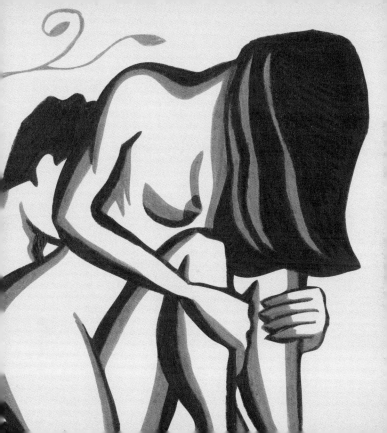

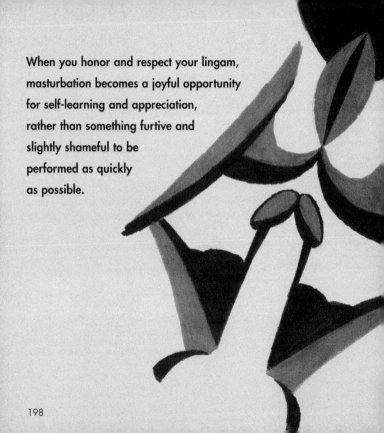

When you honor and respect your lingam, masturbation becomes a joyful opportunity for self-learning and appreciation, rather than something furtive and slightly shameful to be performed as quickly as possible.

The ancient Taoist teachers saw no shame in masturbation—they called it "solo cultivation" and regarded it as an essential part of the process of learning to circulate sexual energy.

A simple shift in perspective
allows you to self-pleasure in a
way that is joyful and sacred.

BRING A MEDITATIVE AWARENESS TO MAKING LOVE
TO YOURSELF. DO IT WITH LOVE, NOT IN ANGER OR
FRUSTRATION. TAKE YOUR TIME, BECOMING AWARE
OF AND LOVING EVERY PART OF YOUR BODY, NOT
JUST YOUR GENITALS.

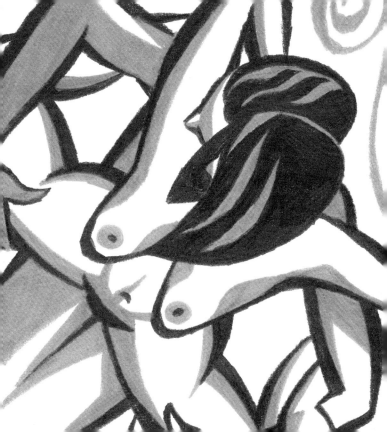

Feel the flow of energy around your body as you engage in unhurried self-pleasuring. Take time to get in touch with your sexual response, to learn about your reaction to touch, and to discover your true inner nature.

Introduce some feminine energy to your self-pleasuring—stroke your entire body, caressing your nipples and inner thighs, and turn your senses inward so that you move from thinking to feeling, taking time to relish every sensation.

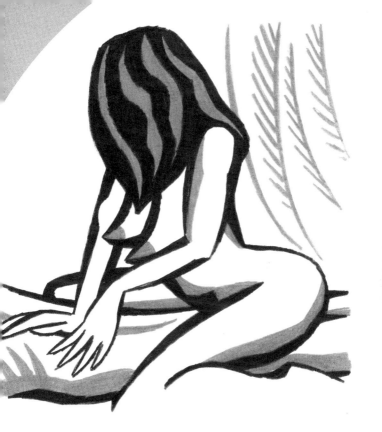

According to legend, the founder of Chinese civilization, the Yellow Emperor, was blessed with three sexual initiators.

These wise women gave him frank advice, which is contained in the classic Chinese erotic texts, and offered explicit instruction on a variety of aspects of lovemaking, especially on how to give a woman the fullest pleasure.

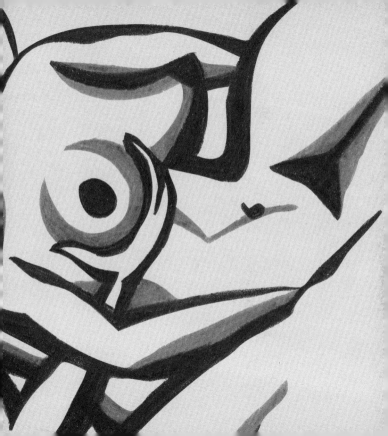

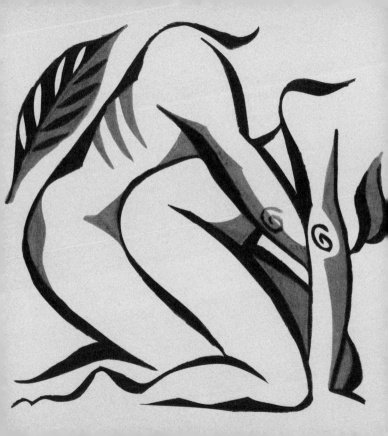

For men who suffer doubts about the size and shape of their lingam, the Yellow Emperor's straight-talking sexual advisor, The Plain Girl, named Su-Nü, has wise words:

A long implement that gets only half hard is not as effective as a short one that grows hard as iron. A short, hard implement that is wielded roughly and without due consideration for the woman's feelings is not nearly as desirable as one used with expertise and careful attention to the woman's responses. As with everything else under Heaven, one should strive for the Golden Mean in achieving the harmony of Yin and Yang.

The Wondrous Discourse of Su-Nü

The Yellow Emperor's advisors told him that women are slower to bring to arousal than men. If a woman is to be fully satisfied in bed, lovemaking must last long enough for her sexual energy to be brought to boiling point.

AND SO MEN WERE TAUGHT TO DELAY, AND EVEN AVOID, EJACULATION.

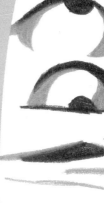

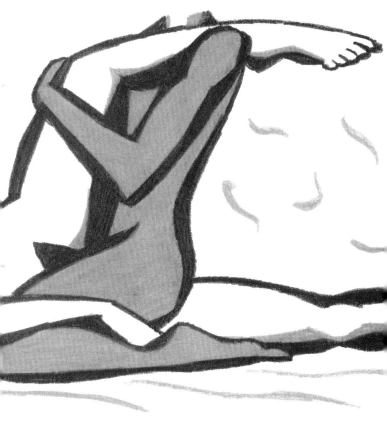

One cannot manage the myriad matters
Of Heaven and Earth,
Unless one stores up energy.
Storing energy means absorbing essence,
And absorbing essence doubles one's power.
Doubling one's power, one acquires a strength
That nothing can overcome.

Tao Te Ching

In sexual intercourse, semen must be regarded as a
most precious substance. By saving it, a man protects
his very life. Whenever he does ejaculate, the loss of
semen must then be compensated by absorbing the
woman essence.

P'eng Tsu

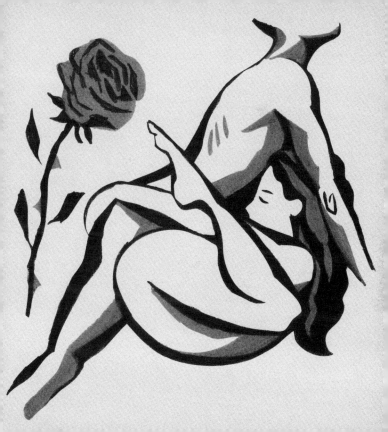

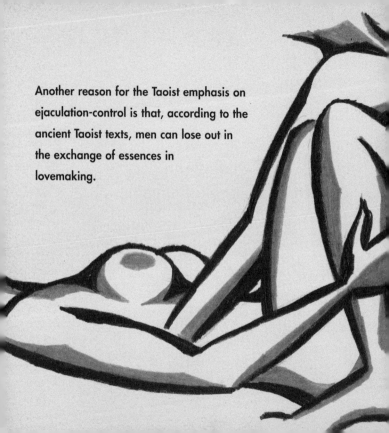

Another reason for the Taoist emphasis on ejaculation-control is that, according to the ancient Taoist texts, men can lose out in the exchange of essences in lovemaking.

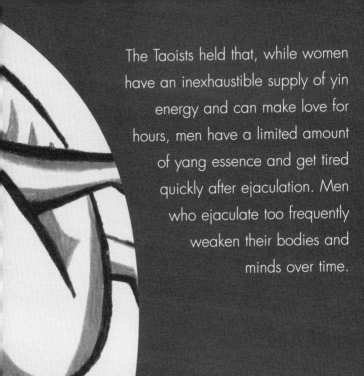

The Taoists held that, while women have an inexhaustible supply of yin energy and can make love for hours, men have a limited amount of yang essence and get tired quickly after ejaculation. Men who ejaculate too frequently weaken their bodies and minds over time.

Once you are in touch with your arousal patterns, start perfecting the art of controlling ejaculation with the suggestions that follow. Then you will be able to voluntarily and consciously adapt your lovemaking to whatever feels right for a particular moment.

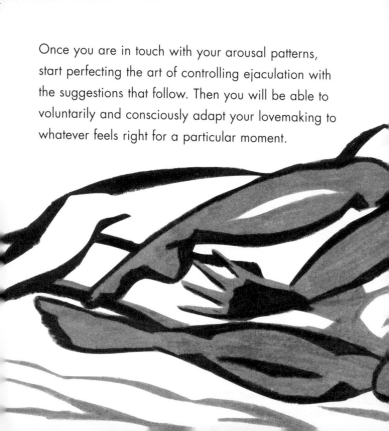

Arousal becomes like a wave, a massive expansion of sexual energy that encompasses a series of peaks of wonderful sensation, rather than one big climax. The longer you can make love, the more healing energy you can generate and circulate, and the greater the likelihood that you will be able to satisfy your lover more completely.

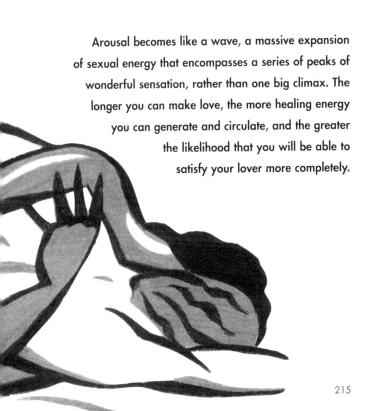

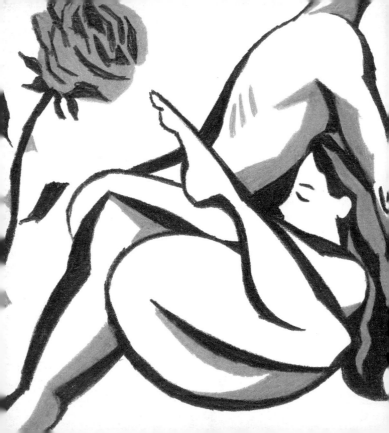

So long as the breath is in
motion, the semen moves also.
When the breath ceases to move,
then the semen remains at rest.

Goraksa Samhita

Different kinds of breathing can help delay ejaculation. When you self-pleasure, experiment with slow, deep breathing as you reach the point of no return, and become used to the cooling-down effect this engenders.

Try a Taoist technique for ejaculation control by developing the PC or "love" muscle (the muscle you feel when you clench to stop a flow of urine).

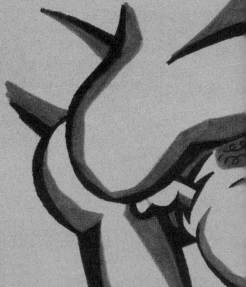

Holding the muscle in a sustained contraction when you approach the point of no return during lovemaking can reverse the flow of sexual energy for long enough to avoid ejaculation.

The perineum press is an effective emergency stop which either you or your lover can put in place without disturbing the flow of lovemaking.

Simply reach around and firmly press the area between the scrotum and anus for a few seconds until arousal has subsided.

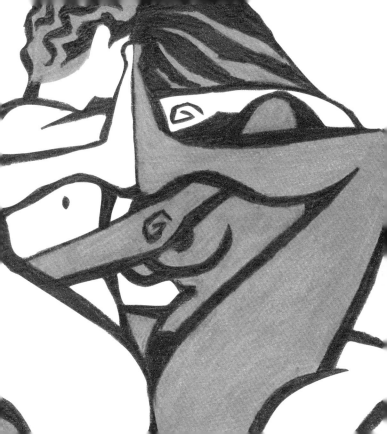

When ejaculation is no longer a goal, your body becomes more relaxed and energy is freed to flow throughout the body in ecstatic, orgasmic joy.

Lovemaking can become an endless journey of pleasure that need no longer come to an abrupt end at the destination of ejaculation.

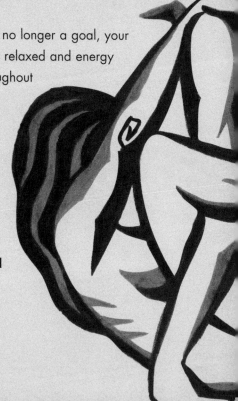

If one engages in sex without emission, then the strength of our chi will be more than sufficient and our bodies at ease. One's hearing will be acute and vision clear. Although exercising self-control and calming the passion, love actually increases and one remains unsatiated. How can this be considered unpleasurable?

P'eng Tsu

There is a brotherhood of Tantrics waiting to be brought to life. This brotherhood will awaken as the end of the Kali Age approaches. Recognizing the potent Female Principle of life, the Brotherhood of Tantra will transform this polluted world. Then at the ecstatic moment when one Age transforms into the next, those faithful followers of the selfless path will reach their goal.

Kaula Tantra

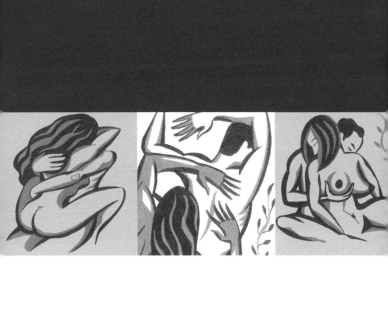

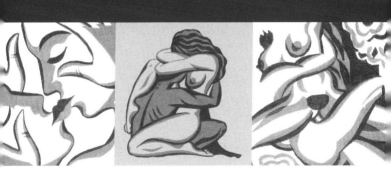

5 TUNING IN

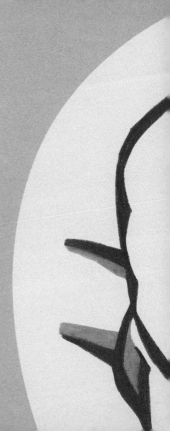

Treat your body, and that of your lover, as a temple, and lovemaking becomes an act of worship.

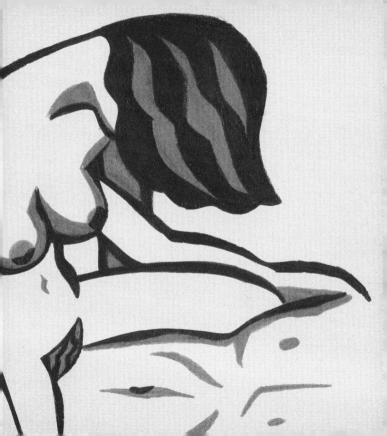

We are all divine beings. When we honor
this aspect of ourselves and our lovers,
sexual relationships are transformed
into sacred partnerships.

At the heart of sacred sex
is surrender to your own
divine potential, and your
connection to your lover
as a fellow spiritual and
sexual being.

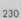

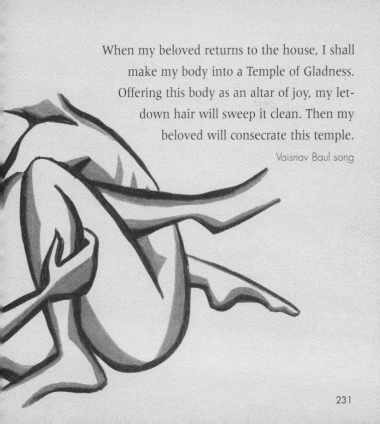

When my beloved returns to the house, I shall make my body into a Temple of Gladness. Offering this body as an altar of joy, my let-down hair will sweep it clean. Then my beloved will consecrate this temple.

Vaisnav Baul song

IN TANTRA, SEXUAL RELATIONSHIPS ARE A
MIRROR OF THE DIVINE PARTNERSHIP BETWEEN
THE PRIMORDIAL COUPLE, SHAKTI AND SHIVA.

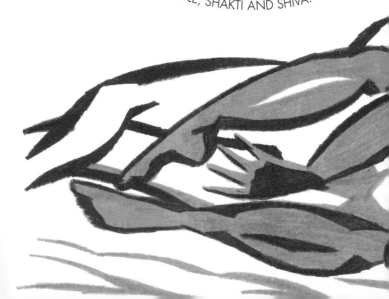

Tantrics call the god and goddess into lovemaking in physical and subtle ways, such as dressing-up, dancing, and meditating, and also aim to make them manifest through posture, breath, and expression.

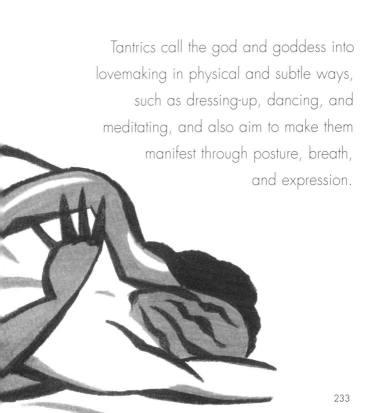

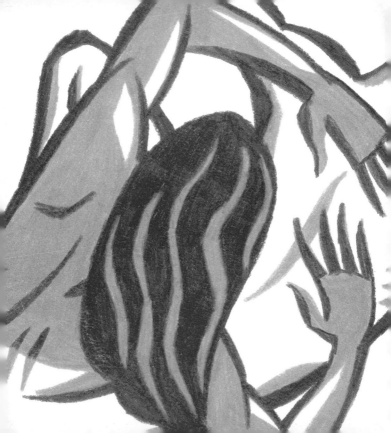

However you choose to
visualize the spiritual energies
within yourself, by acknowledging,
accepting, and embracing them,
you create a strong connection
with your lover on a divine level.

TO EXPLORE AND TOUCH
EACH OTHER THEN BECOMES
AN ACT OF PURE DEVOTION
AND HONORING, SETTING THE
STAGE FOR EXPERIENCING
HEAVEN ON EARTH.

Though familiar with the soft flesh
Of my lover's body,
I cannot measure her depths.

Tsangyang Gyatso, sixth Dalai Lama

To tune into the god- or goddess-
nature of your lover, you need to
rise above the familiar and see
the person with new eyes. By
looking beyond the imperfections
of the human form, you can see
the essence of the other's being
and the radiance within.

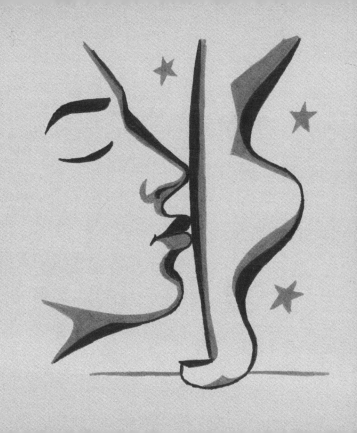

Let a conscious sacred connection
take place long before you touch
each other.

Come to lovemaking with
an attitude of openness and
innocence, appreciating the
inherent beauty of your lover,
and you step into a heartfelt
space of respect and love.

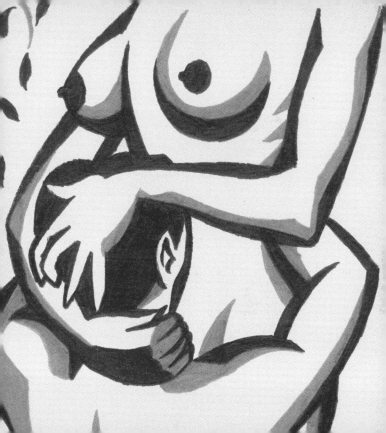

Namaste is a Sanskrit word that means,
'The God in me greets the God in you.
The Spirit in me meets the same Spirit in you.'

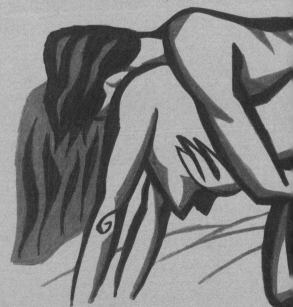

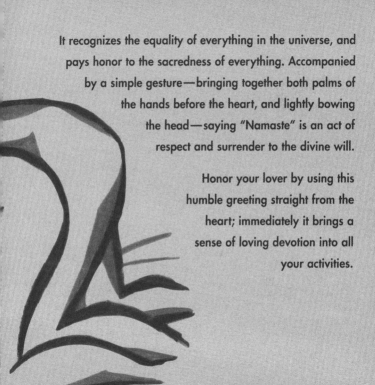

It recognizes the equality of everything in the universe, and pays honor to the sacredness of everything. Accompanied by a simple gesture—bringing together both palms of the hands before the heart, and lightly bowing the head—saying "Namaste" is an act of respect and surrender to the divine will.

Honor your lover by using this humble greeting straight from the heart; immediately it brings a sense of loving devotion into all your activities.

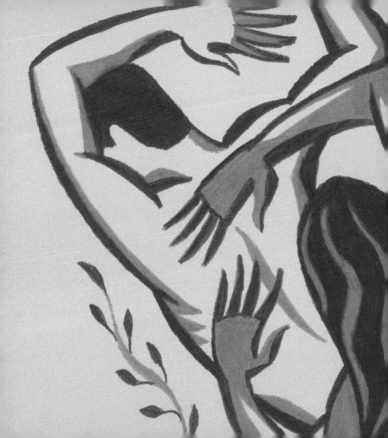

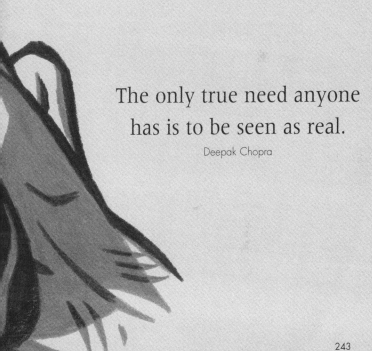

The only true need anyone
has is to be seen as real.

Deepak Chopra

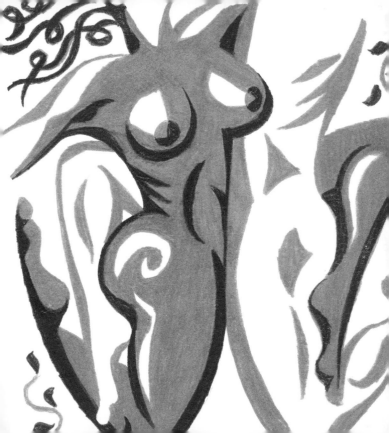

EYE-GAZING IS A SIMPLE BUT
EFFECTIVE WAY TO TUNE INTO YOUR
SOUL-CONNECTION WITH A LOVER.

Sit opposite each other at a
comfortable distance apart and look
steadily into each other's eyes. Still
your mind as well as your gaze,
placing your entire focus on your
lover's presence. Visualize your
partner's eyes as the gateway to
the soul and look deeply within,
tuning into your lover's divine
core. Freely express feelings of
heartfelt love through your eyes.

Turn toward me your azure eyes
that are rich with stars!
For the divine balm of one
delightful glance,
I will lift the veils from love's
most obscure pleasures,
And you shall drowse in endless
dream!

Charles Baudelaire

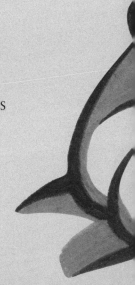

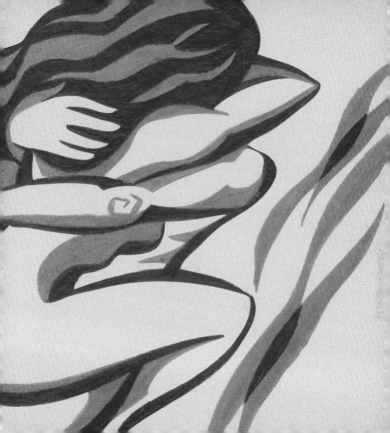

We live lives, even our sex lives, in a rush, hurrying from one sensation to the next. With the mind always racing on to the next thought, it is all too easy to forget to experience the here and now.

Stop, and be still!

Truly connecting before sex means bringing awareness into every action, taking time to appreciate the presence of your lover, and being fully present in each unfolding moment together.

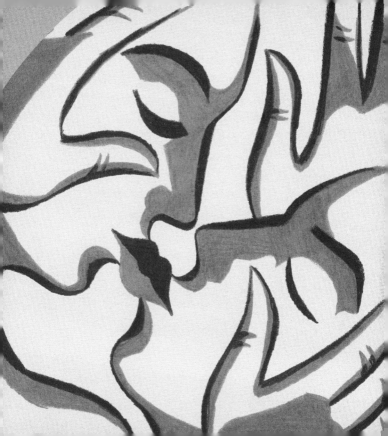

Spiritual sex isn't about having the most lithe body—
we all have imperfections—instead it's about
understanding that the body is a vehicle for the spirit.

Spiritual sex isn't about fancy postures or
techniques—you can learn all the techniques
in the manual, yet still employ them with
a cold heart.

True spiritual sex happens when you engage your open mind, body, and spirit with your lover's mind, body, and spirit, fully in the moment. For this you need to generate awareness.

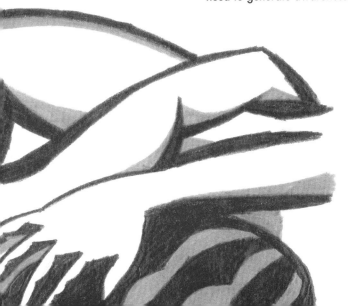

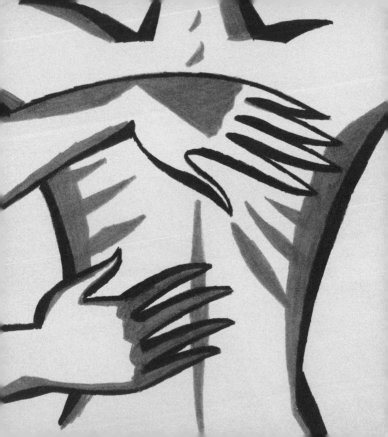

Pausing to tune in to each other before lovemaking invites a different quality of awareness. Do this and find yourselves magically in flow with the vibrations of each other's subtle body, becoming aware of the presence and movement of the other person's energy.

Heart-, forehead-, and fingertip-touching are tuning-in exercises from the Sufi tradition, the mystical path of Islam, and create a wonderfully intimate connection.

Sit cross-legged opposite each other with knees touching. Both place your right palm on the other person's heart. Now place your left hand over your lover's right hand, covering it. Gaze into each other's eyes and breathe in harmony. Feel the love connection between you, streaming out of your hearts and back in through your hands.

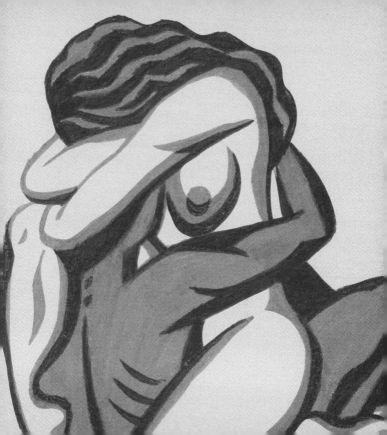

Still in the same position, touch foreheads together. Close your eyes and enjoy the feeling of closeness and intimacy.

Try complementary breathing: as you exhale, visualize your breath entering your lover's third-eye chakra (see page 99). Your partner inhales, picturing the breath coming from your third eye, and exhales it back as you inhale again.

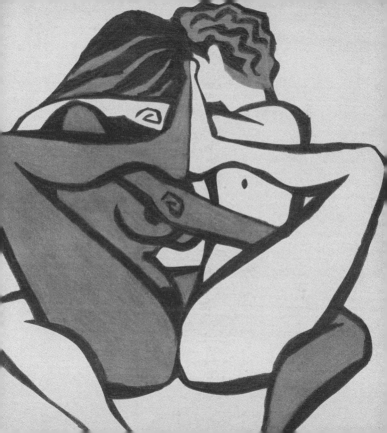

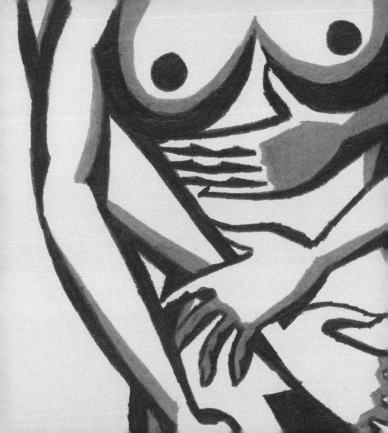

Establishing the connection between you by touching fingertips can be fun.

Either rest your fingertips lightly against each other, or play with increasing the pressure on each fingertip in turn, as if playing an arpeggio against your lover's fingers. Center your awareness on the sensation in each fingertip as you feel the energy buzz and circulate.

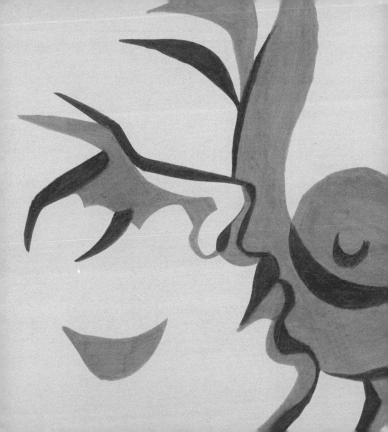

WORSHIP RITUALS CAN HELP FOCUS THE
MIND AND ENHANCE INTERNAL FEELINGS
OF DEVOTION. KNOWN AS PUJA IN
HINDUISM, DEVOTIONAL RITUALS ARE
COMMON IN TEMPLES AND
SYMBOLIZE THE OFFERING OF AN
ENTIRE SENSUAL WORLD.

Bring all the senses alive in your
worship of your lover as an
embodiment of the divine, and share
rituals by bathing, offering gifts of
flowers, ringing bells, or burning
incense before lovemaking.

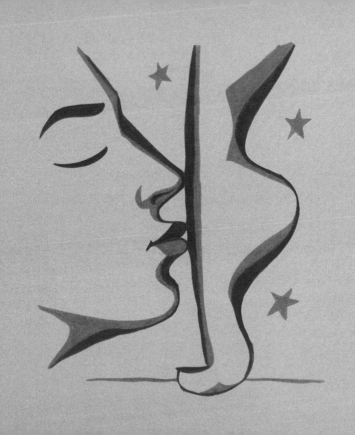

Having seen one's partner as a god or goddess, one naturally feels a sense of devotion. At this point there is no need for elaborate instructions, as love play spontaneously becomes the sport of deities. Every gesture becomes an act of worship, every sigh and word of love becomes a prayer, and gazing into the lover's eyes becomes a one-pointed meditation.

Miranda Shaw

Honoring the sacred connection between you and your lover sends ripples into your lives far beyond the time you spend making love.

Carry a sense of loving devotion into all interactions with your partner, and see how your relationship takes on a new light. In doing this, you encourage an appreciation and respect that puts everyday angst and squabbles into perspective.

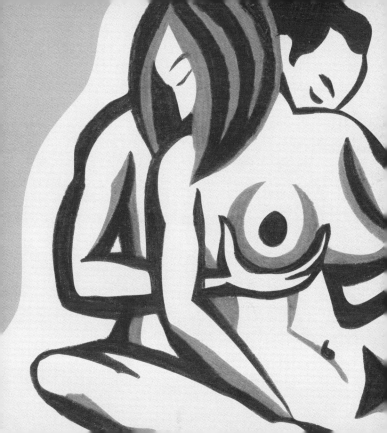

Becoming god and goddess to each other allows you to let go of the self you usually show to the world and reconnect with your true nature.

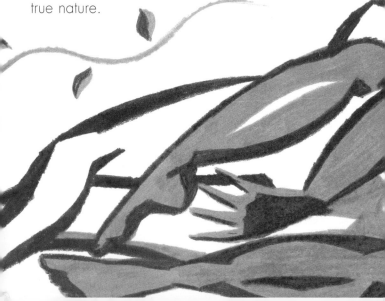

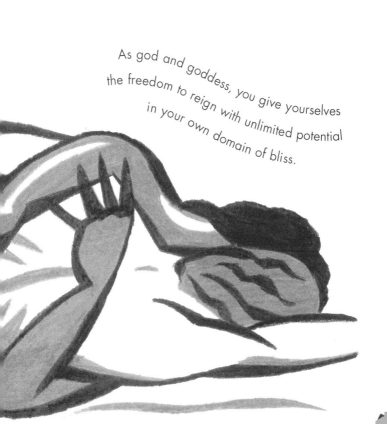

As god and goddess, you give yourselves
the freedom to reign with unlimited potential
in your own domain of bliss.

TANTRA TEACHES THAT BECAUSE WHAT IS NOT
HERE IS NOT FOUND ANYWHERE, WE SHOULD
ENJOY WHAT IS HERE.

SO SHED THE CARES OF DAYTIME LIFE ALONG
WITH YOUR CLOTHES, AND BECOME ENCHANTED,
MYSTIFIED, AND DELIGHTED WITH EACH OTHER.

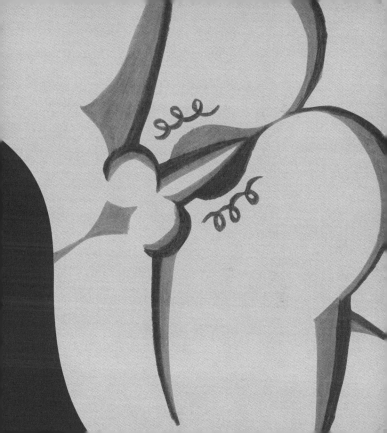

The man sees the woman as a goddess,
The woman sees the man as a god.
By joining the diamond scepter and lotus,
They should make offerings to each other.
There is no worship apart from this.

Candamaharosana Tantra

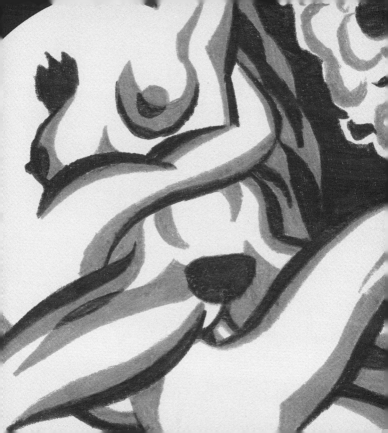

Mantras are sacred sounds that, when uttered, create a unique vibrational energy. They are used as a tool to aid awareness in meditation.

Introduce sacred sound into your lovemaking by approaching it as a kind of ecstatic meditation and chant a mantra with your lover before sex; it helps to create harmonious vibrations between you, and keeps you focused in the moment.

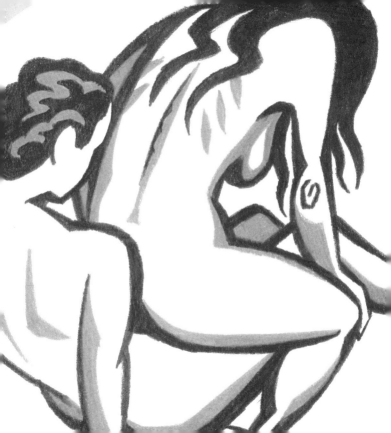

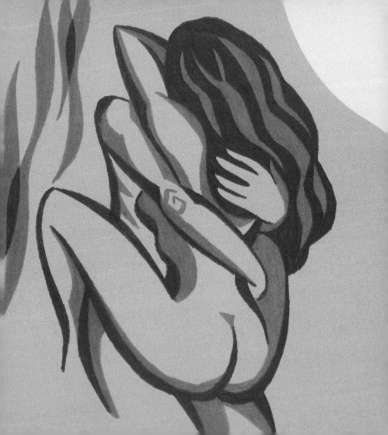

THE SOUND OF THE BREATH AND
THE HEARTBEAT ARE OUR MOST
PERSONAL MANTRAS.

The "supreme" mantra,
Om, from which all other sounds
derive, is said to be the sound of
the universe humming.

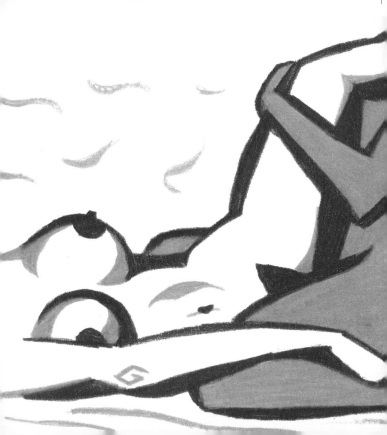

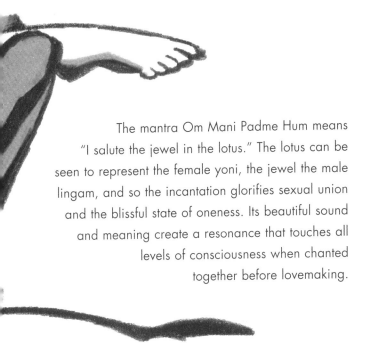

The mantra Om Mani Padme Hum means "I salute the jewel in the lotus." The lotus can be seen to represent the female yoni, the jewel the male lingam, and so the incantation glorifies sexual union and the blissful state of oneness. Its beautiful sound and meaning create a resonance that touches all levels of consciousness when chanted together before lovemaking.

Try creating your own mantra that has a special meaning for you. It could be a positive affirmation, such as "we are one," or simply a powerful vibrational resonance of pure sound.

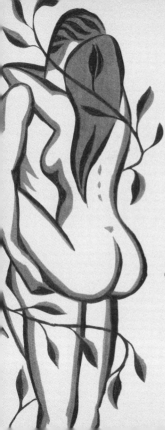

Actions dance to the rhythm of a mantra—a slow mantra will promote calm and relaxation, a fast mantra can help generate energy.

Listen to the cries of pleasure
you and your lover release
during lovemaking.

WHAT DO YOU HEAR?

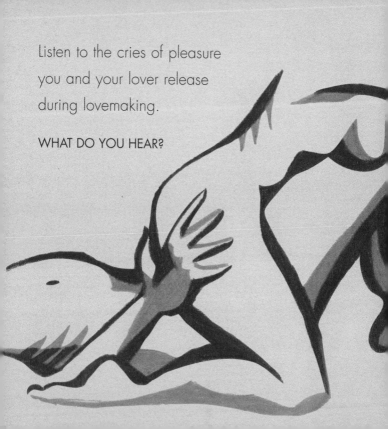

Value these sounds as the natural
and unself-conscious expression
of the moment, the sound of
souls singing out in ecstasy.

COULD THIS BE YOUR MANTRA?

When we make love with spiritual awareness, we open up the body's energy centers in ways that sometimes feel uncomfortable. The Tantrics use psychic-protection techniques to encourage a feeling of safety as the heart and body open.

BY CONCENTRATING CONSCIOUSNESS ON VARIOUS PARTS OF THE BODY, OPENINGS ARE "SEALED" TO PROVIDE PROTECTION FROM NEGATIVE ENERGIES OUTSIDE AND LOSS OF ENERGY WITHIN. THIS ACTION ALSO CREATES AN EROTIC, POLARIZED ENERGY CIRCUIT THAT OPENS THE HEART CENTER.

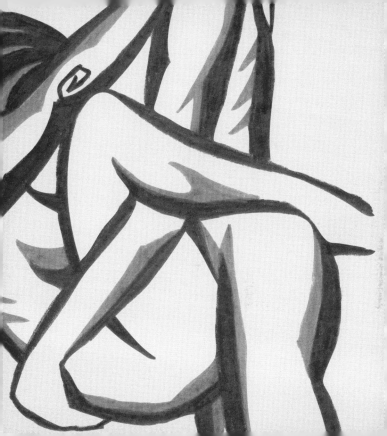

The establishment of a field of psychic protection should be part of every love-act, and is ideally suited to foreplay. Many couples experience sudden and unaccountable feelings of fear or loss during particularly passionate love-making. Simple psychic protection will prevent this.

Nik Douglas

With the first two fingers, touch the partner's head, forehead, eyes, throat, earlobes, breasts, upper arms, heart, navel, thighs, feet, and sexual organ. Charge these places with the vital energy of transformation.

Yogini Tantra

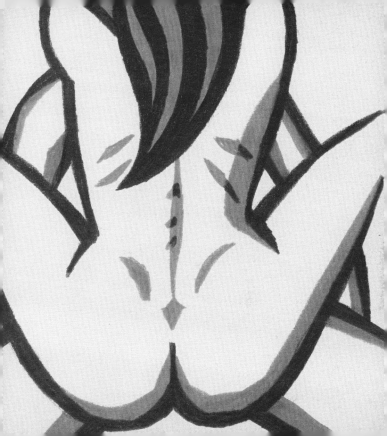

NYASA, OR "PLACING," IS A WARM AND INTIMATE PSYCHIC-PROTECTION RITUAL TO SHARE BEFORE LOVEMAKING.

Sit naked, opposite each other, and hold hands. Eye-gaze to tune in to each other (see page 245). With a gentle touch of the fingertips, touch each other simultaneously on the palms, feet, genitals, navel, breasts, lips, earlobes, eyelids, and third eye. Repeating a mantra as you anoint each area can aid concentration. You could try breathing softly as you touch, or adding a gentle kiss each time.

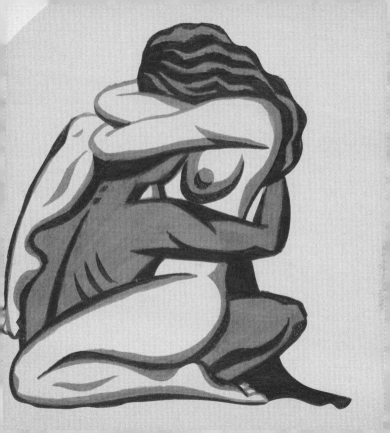

Touching each part of your
body, I also touch my body
and I realize we are One.

From the Sri Chakra Yantra ceremony

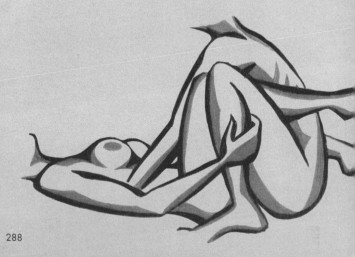

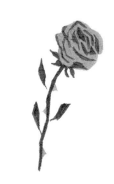

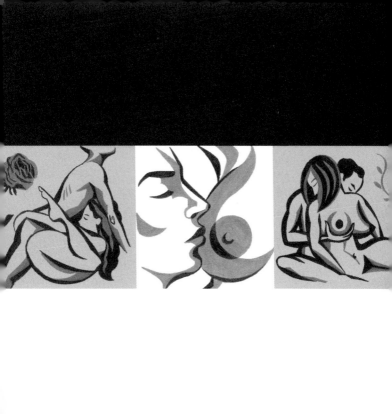

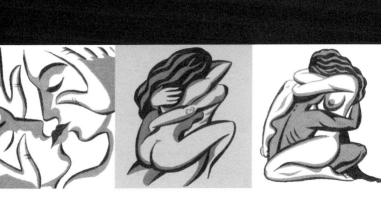

6 ENERGY **CONNECTIONS**

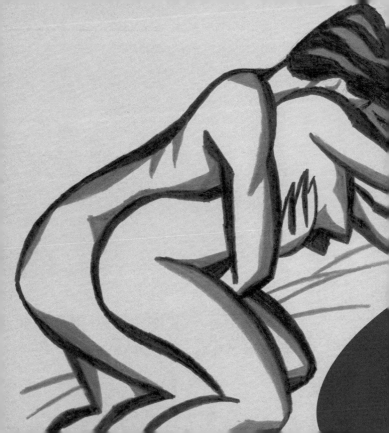

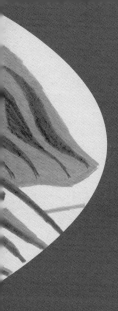

The natural intercoursing of sexual energy between lovers is the raw material that sexual alchemists turn into spiritual gold.

When we create and unify life-energy during lovemaking, we learn the secret of uniting spirit with flesh and thus heaven with earth.

The vital essence courses through
the body in invisible currents
of zigzag patterns. These are
like the waves of sound,
in an upward direction
like flames of fire, and
in a downward direction
like rivulets of water.

Sushruta Samhita

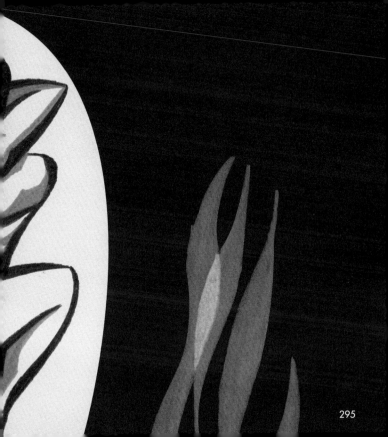

Most of us are only aware of sexual energy in one area of the body—the genital and pelvic region—and in a rush to intensify sensations here and reach the goal of orgasm, we tense up.

By softening instead of tensing, we can yield to the movement of sexual energy upward and outward, and direct it to every part of ourselves. This allows the orgasmic sensation to rise in waves of pure ecstasy throughout the body.

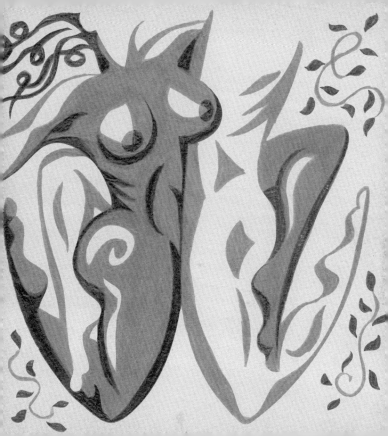

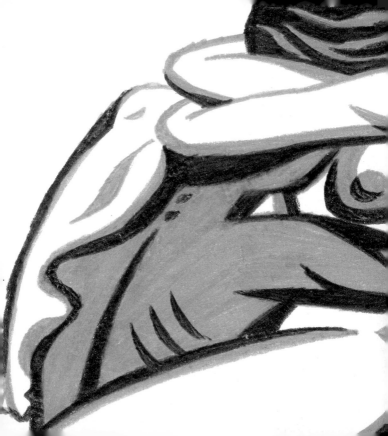

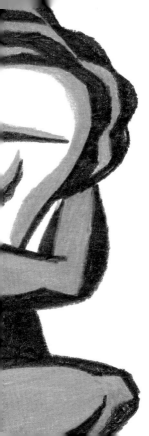

Softening the body, stilling the mind, and opening up to the energy currents flowing within, we create the conditions for sexual magic to unfold.

Spiritual sex is slow sex.

No longer rushing toward orgasm, we transform lovemaking into a series of moments of pleasure in the "now." As well as freeing the flow of sexual energy, this makes sex a voyage of discovery, connection, and growth.

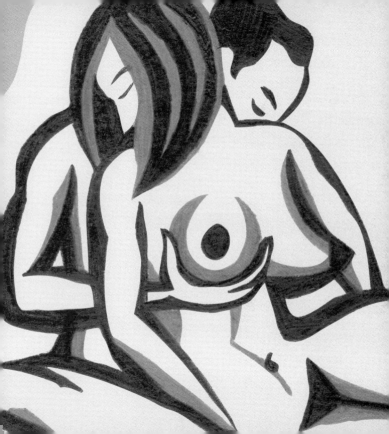

The breath is a powerful tool with which to expand awareness and relax into the sensation of free-flowing energy.

When a couple practice Tantric love, their Shakti and Shiva principles unite with each other and within themselves. At the same time there is a convergence and synchronization of their breaths. Their life-forces merge into a single vortex of pure ecstatic energy and an exchange of physical and subtle energies takes place.

Nik Douglas

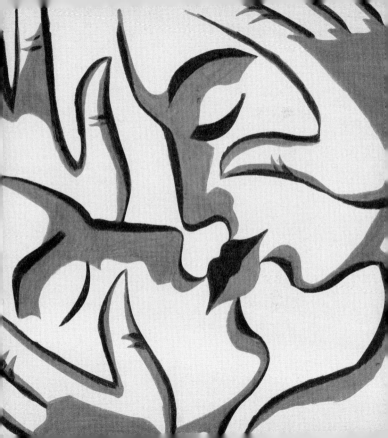

BREATH IS LIFE, AND AWARENESS
OF BREATH IS POWER. TANTRICS
AND TAOISTS UNDERSTOOD
THIS, AND DEVISED
BREATHING SCIENCES—
PRANAYAMA AND CHI
GONG—TO WORK
WITH THE POWER
OF BREATH.

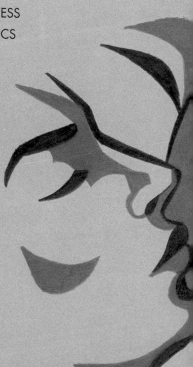

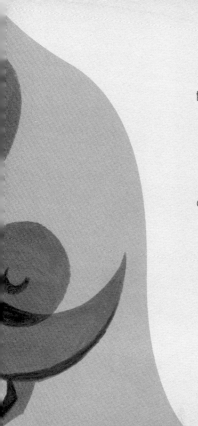

Both practices teach that
through correct breathing
we draw in the cosmic
power of the universe.
Natural breathing drives
and directs vital life-force
through the body's web
of energy channels.

As babies, we all breathed naturally, but few people carry the habit of easy, deep breathing into adulthood. We tend to take shallow breaths into the upper chest, using only a fraction of the lungs' capacity.

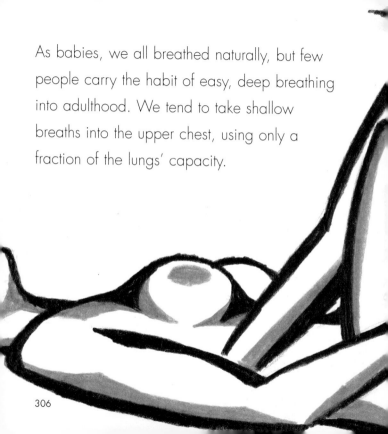

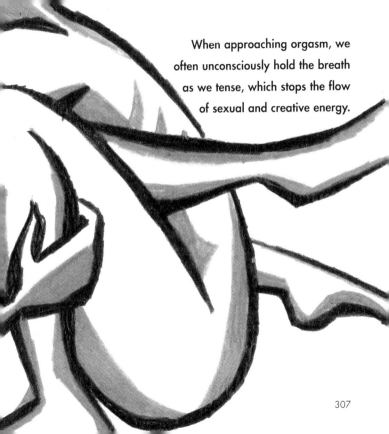

When approaching orgasm, we often unconsciously hold the breath as we tense, which stops the flow of sexual and creative energy.

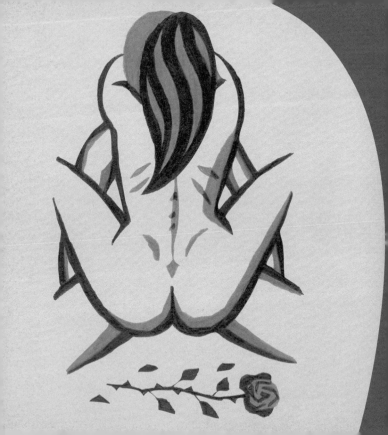

Try taking a few moments of stillness to
become aware of your breath.

Sit comfortably with a straight spine and close your eyes.
Breathe in your regular way through your nose, and focus
on the passage of air through the body as you inhale and
exhale completely. Warm your hands and place them just
beneath your ribs. Feel the rise and fall of your
diaphragm as the breath comes and goes. As you take
smooth, slow breaths, fill yourself from abdomen to chest,
and then empty yourself from abdomen to chest. Breathe
in this way for up to ten minutes.

How different do your body
and mind feel now?

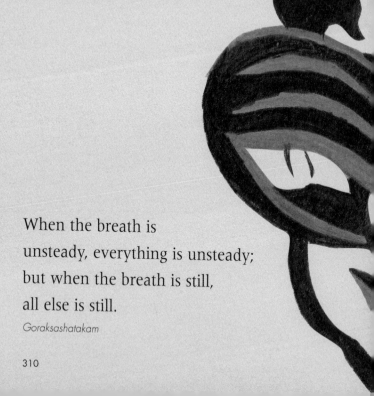

When the breath is
unsteady, everything is unsteady;
but when the breath is still,
all else is still.

Goraksashatakam

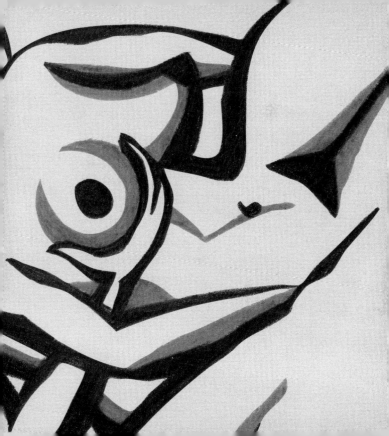

Deep, slow breathing is the cornerstone
breath of conscious sex.

Breathe deeply to maintain a calm and meditative
state of mind in the midst of a maelstrom of sensations.

Breathe deeply when you need to cool down, when excitement takes you to the edge of the precipice, but you feel as if you want to carry on forever.

Breathe deeply in tune with your lover to nourish your sense of connection with each other.

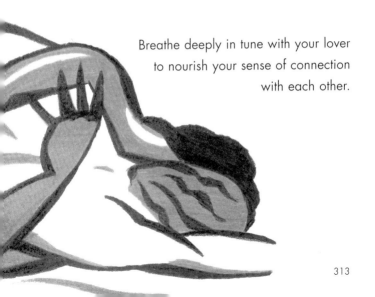

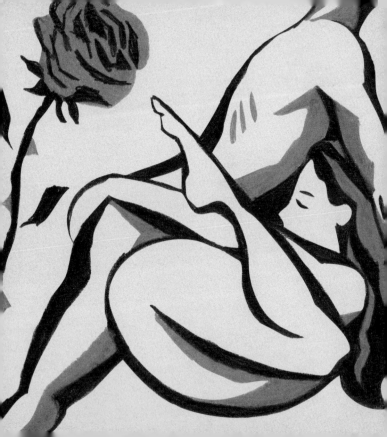

SOMETIMES WE NEED FAST, HARD BREATHING, TOO.

Breathe quickly with intensity for a heating
effect that energizes and arouses.

Try panting rapidly from the stomach, with an
open mouth, when you feel yourself holding
your breath during high states of arousal.

Sharing breathing is a powerfully intimate form of nonverbal communication.

It is simple to learn, but takes you and your lover on a profound journey together, as you float on your breath connection to a place of deep intimacy and peace.

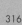

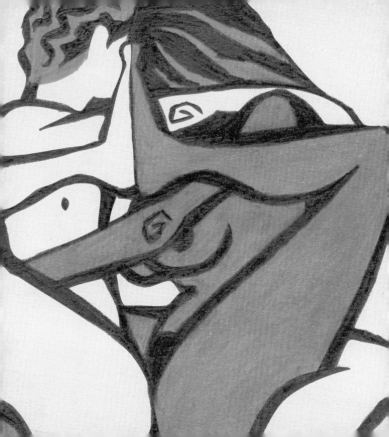

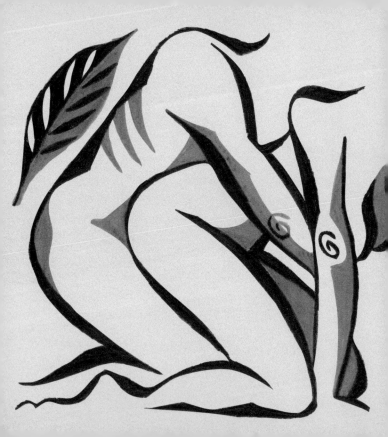

To synchronize your breathing with your lover's, simply match your breath so that you both inhale and exhale at the same time.

Breathe in tune with each other to enhance the sense of connection between you, and to create a peaceful rhythm to your lovemaking.

As you breathe, imagine drawing energy up from your root chakra, raising it through each chakra as you do so (see pages 88–100). Placing a hand on each chakra as you reach it can help you maintain awareness.

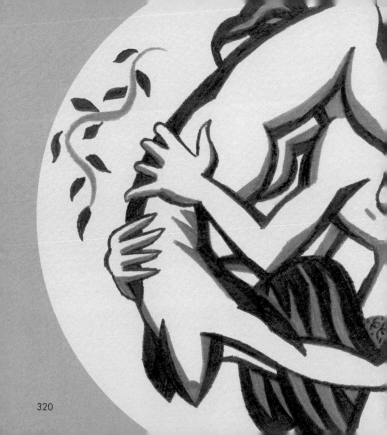

Complementary breathing forms the Tantric "binding breath" in which lovers absorb and bestow each other's life-force with every breath.

Settle your breathing together, then as you exhale, your lover inhales, and vice versa, setting up a circular pattern.

To create a circle of erotic energy, imagine breathing in through your root chakra and out through your heart center, as your lover inhales that breath in through the heart and out through the root chakra.

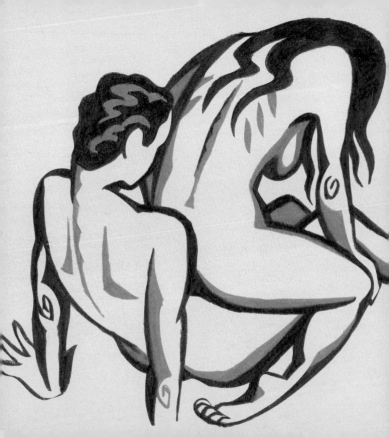

Combine breath awareness with movement to charge the body with energy.

PELVIC BOUNCING IS A SIMPLE BUT EFFECTIVE WAY TO ENERGIZE THE ROOT CHAKRA.

Lie comfortably on your back with knees bent. Breathe deeply, and make sure your shoulders and neck are relaxed. Raise your pelvis up from the floor and start to "bounce" it up and down. Feel the energy streaming through your pelvis, and, with each breath, visualize it moving up the body.

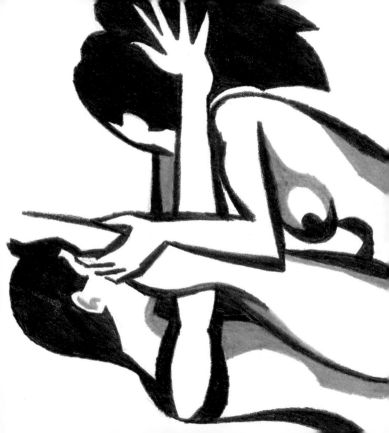

To get a tangible sense of the power
within you, try building a ball of energy.

Close your eyes and rub your hands together
quickly until they feel very warm. Now take
them apart and see if you can sense a
subtle energetic presence between
your palms. Feel what happens as
you move them slowly together
(but not touching) and apart.

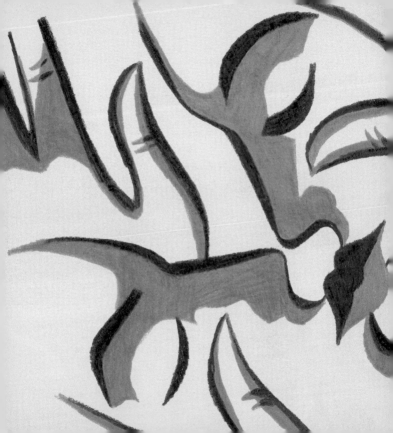

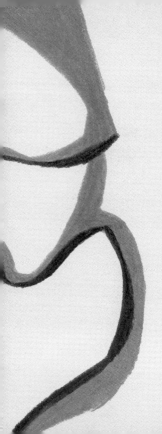

Try juggling balls of energy
with your lover.

Once you have both made a ball of
energy (see page 325), hold your
hands so that your palms face the
other person's, but do not touch. Feel
the energy flow between you as you
move your hands closer together and
further apart. Link your breathing
together with the movement to
increase the intensity of the sensation.

Visualization and breath-work offer a powerful way to create intense energy circuits with the whole body before or during sex.

As you sit or lie with bodies entwined, the first partner inhales, visualizing energy entering the body through the mouth, nose, eyes, and ears. Picture this energy moving downward, then, as you exhale, direct it out through your root chakra.

The other partner then inhales, picturing the same energy entering the body through the root chakra and directing it upward. As the energy rises, it increases in intensity: imagine it leaving the body through the mouth, nose, eyes, and ears with the exhalation.

Repeat the circular pattern of inhalation and exhalation, with the first partner inhaling again.

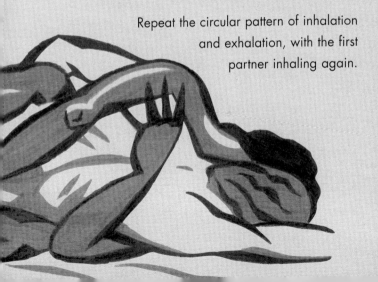

Lovemaking generates huge amounts of powerful energy. When this becomes too chaotic and leaves the head spinning, you need to reestablish your connection with the earth.

Knowing how to ground energy is as important as being able to raise and move it. Once grounded, we are brought to rest, solid and still, as one integrated flow of energy.

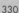

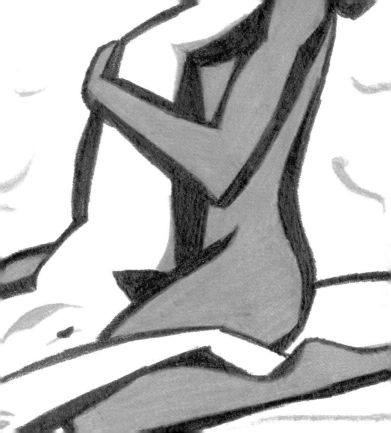

BECOME
A TREE,
ROOTED
IN THE
EARTH.

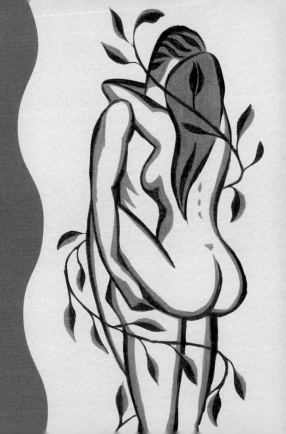

Stop and take a few full, deep breaths. Stand solidly, toes spread out to achieve fullest contact with the ground. Sense the weight of your body and the pull of gravity. Feel roots extending down from your feet, pulling you into the earth. Visualize your body as the tree's solid trunk, holding firm against the push and pull of the energy around you. Hold, being aware of each inhalation and exhalation, for a few minutes.

SIMPLE GROUNDING STRETCHES HELP
EASE OUT ANY PARTS OF THE BODY
THAT MIGHT FEEL TIRED AFTER A
SESSION OF PASSION.

From a standing position, rise onto
your toes, then lower your heels
to the ground, bending your knees.
Feel yourself push against gravity,
then sink into it. Hold, then carefully
come back to standing straight.

Taking a shower or eating some light
food are great "earthing" activities to
share with your lover after sex.

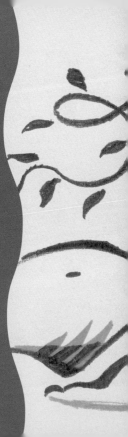

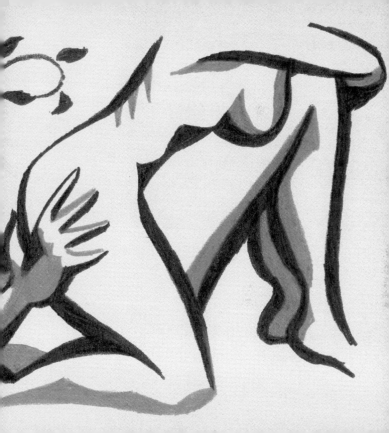

The perfume from her narcissus causes my
bud to sprout, sealing our love pact.

The delicate fragrance
of the flower of eros,

A waterborne nymph,
she engulfs me in love play,

Night after night, by the emerald sea,
under the azure sky.

Zen monk Ikkyu

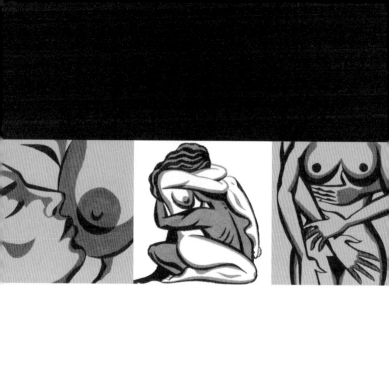

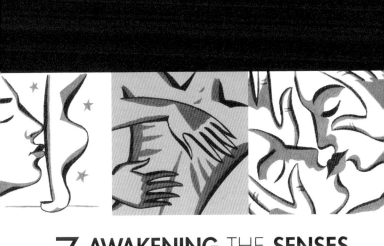

7 AWAKENING THE SENSES

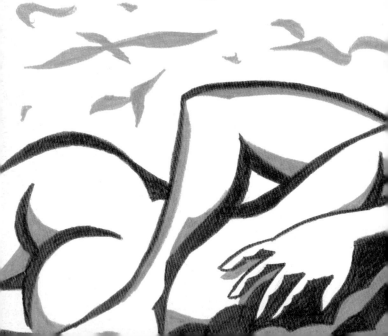

In spiritual sex, it's the journey that matters,
not the destination.

This new perspective shifts the emphasis of sex. We move from a rush for climax into the exploration of total intimacy and sensual pleasure that is making love.

Foreplay is no longer the prelude to the excitement to come, but a vital time of expansion that enables sex to become a truly fulfilling experience for body, mind, and spirit.

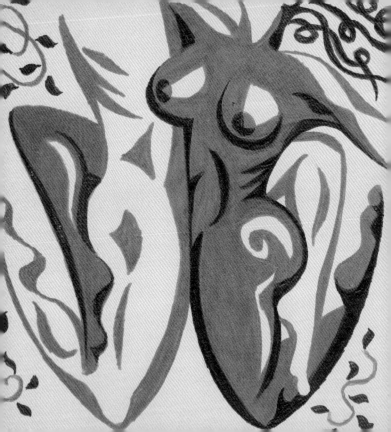

When one enters
    the palace of the sense organs
Experiencing abundant delights
This very world attains
The singular taste of spiritual ecstasy.

Sahajayoginicinta

When we arouse all the senses as tools of
passion and transformation, we eroticize the
whole body and open it up to sensitivity
beyond the scope of ordinary sensory
perceptions. By moving the spotlight away from
the obvious sexual organs, we stop limiting our
knowledge of what it is to be fully sexual.

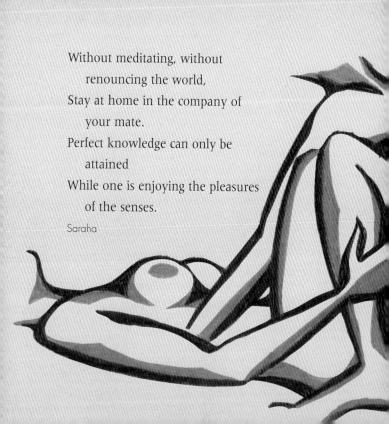

Without meditating, without
    renouncing the world,
Stay at home in the company of
    your mate.
Perfect knowledge can only be
    attained
While one is enjoying the pleasures
    of the senses.

Saraha

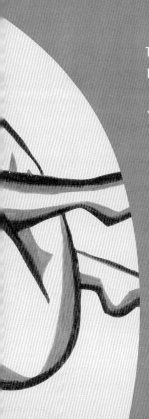

TRY BLINDFOLDING YOUR LOVER, TO
ENLIVEN HIS OR HER OTHER SENSES
AND DEEPEN THE TRUST BETWEEN
YOU. THEN TAKE HIM OR HER ON A
JOURNEY OF THE SENSES,
AWAKENING TASTE, SOUND,
SMELL, AND TOUCH
CONSECUTIVELY.

Tease your lover's taste buds with bite-sized morsels of delicious, sweet-smelling foods—juicy mango pieces, peeled grapes, and cubes of Turkish delight are perfect.

Let your partner enjoy the scent of each morsel before slowly brushing it over the lips and tongue and slipping it into the mouth. Drip tiny ice cubes into the mouth to refresh the palate between flavors.

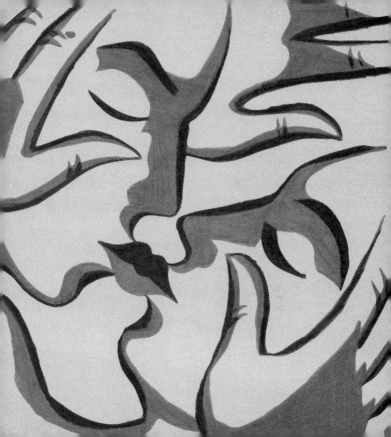

With your lover still blindfolded, awaken his or her sense of smell with wafts of incense, evocative scents, essential oils, and fresh flowers. Intersperse musky, sensual scents, such as jasmine and ylang-ylang, with zesty aromas like peppermint or orange. And don't forget how powerfully arousing the smell of your own skin can be...

"Delicious is the smell of your fragrance,"
whispers the bride in the Old Testament's
Song of Songs **to her divine lover.**
"Your name is perfume
poured out."

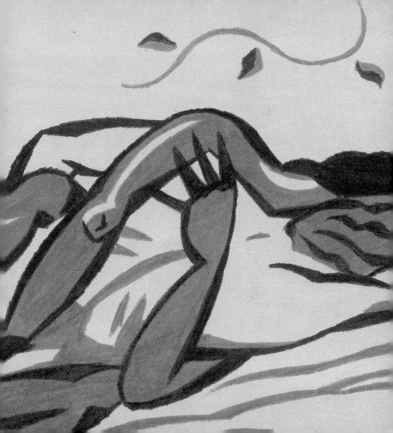

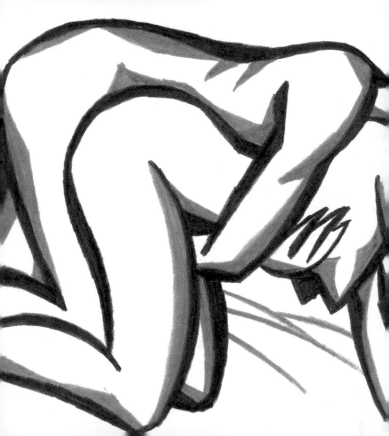

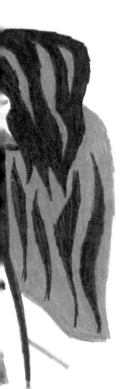

To awaken your lover's sense of sound, whisper and murmur in both ears, and make harmonious noises in different areas of the room. Use bells, gongs, or finger cymbals; alternatively, play short excerpts of beautiful music.

Gently massage your lover's ears, and then nibble, lick, and suck them to create an erotic cocktail of sound and touch.

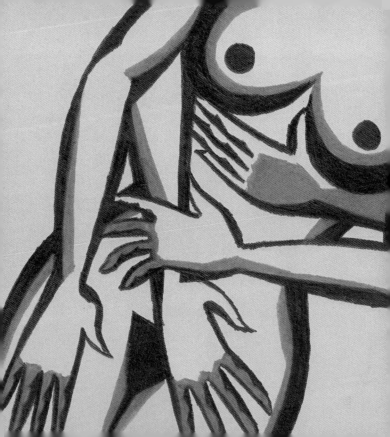

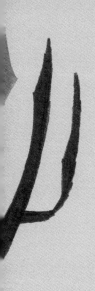

Form is perceived by the eye; sound is heard by the ear; smell is experienced by the nose; taste is experienced by the tongue; objects are felt by the body and the mind experiences pleasure and so forth. These, which are worthy of adoration, should be served.

Hevajra Tantra

Dissolve your whole body into vision, so
to become seeing, seeing, seeing...
Rumi

After awakening taste, sound, and smell,
remove your lover's blindfold and gaze
deeply into each other's eyes, as if seeing
your partner for the first time. As Rumi
advises, bring an awareness of every part
of the body into your focus and soul-gaze,
and sink completely into each other's eyes.

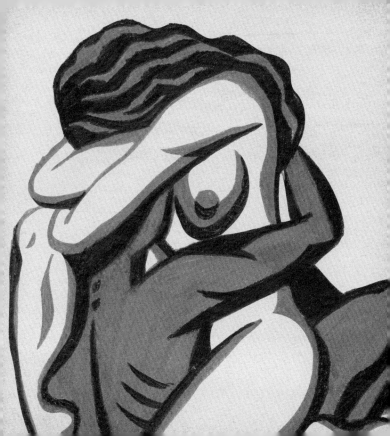

Touch is always mutual. We can see without being seen, hear without being heard, and smell without emitting a scent. But no one can touch without being touched. Whether playful, arousing, relaxing, or healing, touch is something we all need to give and receive.

BRING YOUR SENSE OF TOUCH
INTO PLAY TO INITIATE A SILENT,
INTIMATE CONVERSATION
WITH YOUR LOVER'S BODY.

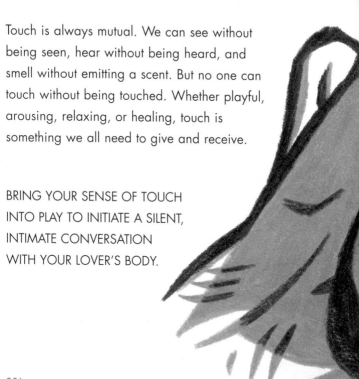

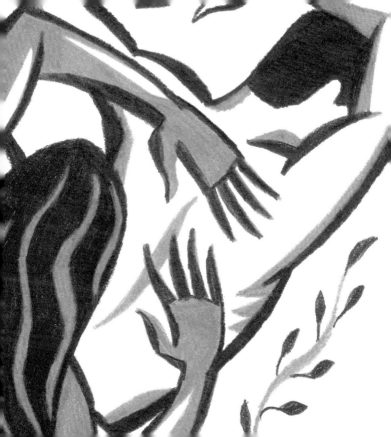

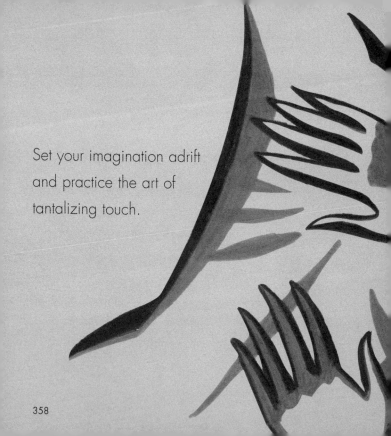

Set your imagination adrift
and practice the art of
tantalizing touch.

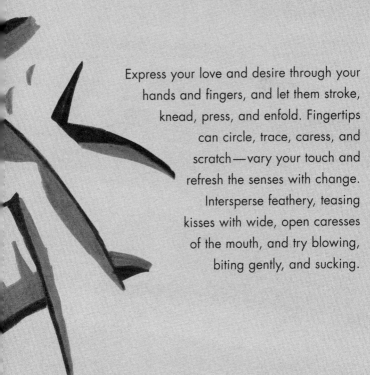

Express your love and desire through your hands and fingers, and let them stroke, knead, press, and enfold. Fingertips can circle, trace, caress, and scratch—vary your touch and refresh the senses with change. Intersperse feathery, teasing kisses with wide, open caresses of the mouth, and try blowing, biting gently, and sucking.

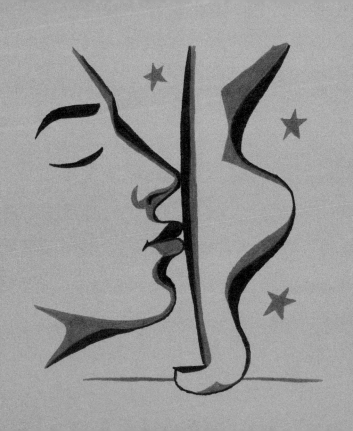

Don't forget to use your feet and toes—
feel the difference in skin textures as you
run your feet along your partner's calves and
use your toes to gently tweak or circle nipples.

**Use long hair to stroke and trail across the skin, or to
trace the outline of lips, nipples, and navel.**

Keep different sensual materials on hand,
such as feathers, silk, and velvet, to stroke
and run along the skin.

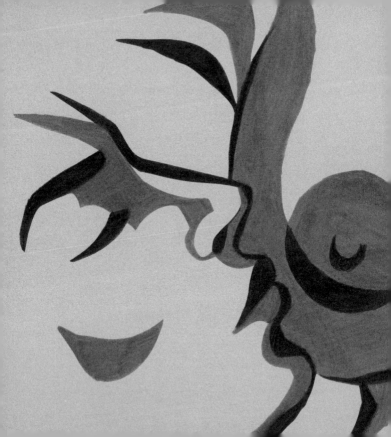

Erogenous zones are our own personal hot spots—places where we are easily aroused with a caress or a kiss.

The sexual organs are our most obvious erogenous zones, but, according to the ancient Tantrics and Taoists, the entire body is ripe for arousal. Once awakened by the mind (the most powerful erogenous zone of all), energy is freed to circulate and create a whole-body sensual experience.

Take time to find your lover's unexpected sweet spots. It could be the earlobes, toes, back of the knee, or elbow crease. Or all of these!

Explore and experiment, playfully stimulating different areas in different ways—stroking, scratching, kissing, sucking—until you find the spot and the touch that makes your lover shiver with pleasure.

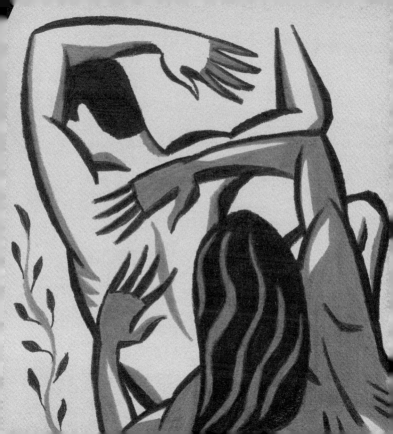

Take it slowly! There's no goal to hurry to,
only the pleasure of the journey.

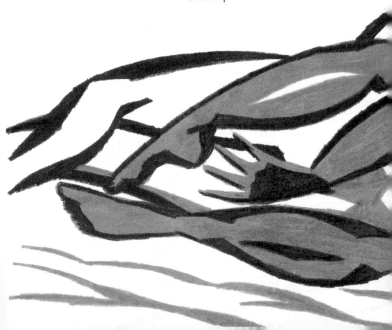

The most powerful erogenous zone is the mind—
stir the imagination and the body will respond.

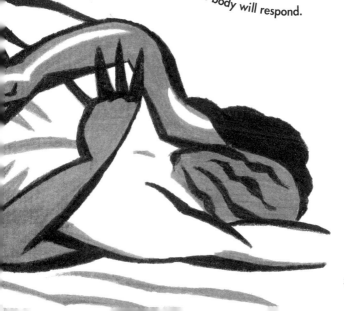

The kiss is the
gateway to bliss.

Kama Sutra

A humid kiss is better
than a hurried coitus.

Arab proverb

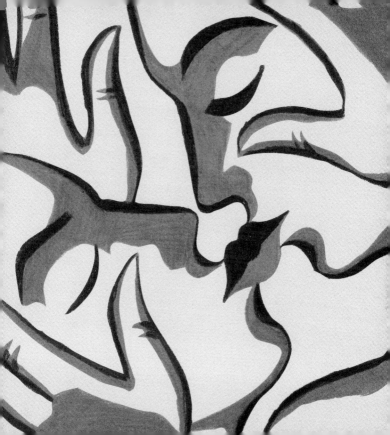

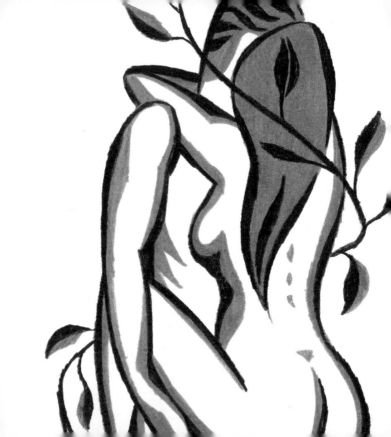

Can you remember the last time you spent more than a few minutes simply kissing your lover?

Kissing is one of the finer arts of love that is often sadly neglected. In established relationships, we might not take time to indulge in the long, erotic kisses enjoyed during courtship, and during sex such kisses may be relegated to the beginning of foreplay, if included at all.

Yet mouths and tongues have the power to arouse intense sexual energy, and passionate kissing is one of the most intimate acts we can share with a lover.

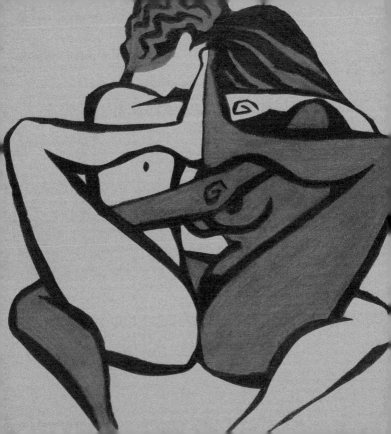

The Taoists and Tantrics fully understood the erotic power of the kiss. Taoists placed deep kissing second only to the act of love itself, while Tantrics taught that a woman's upper lip is connected by a special nerve channel directly to the clitoris. Kissing and nibbling the lips awakens this channel and allows powerful erotic energy to circulate.

EXPERIENCE THIS EROTIC ENERGY WHEN YOU KISS— THE MOUTH AND TONGUE ARE POTENT ENERGY TERMINALS, AND DEEP, PASSIONATE KISSING CREATES A CIRCUIT FOR THE FLOW OF SEXUAL ENERGY THAT TINGLES THROUGHOUT THE BODY.

The tongue is the main switch for the chi flowing in your microcosmic orbit. Whenever you kiss deeply or lick her, your life energy flows into her, and hers into you. A power tongue is like a magic wand, sprinkling bliss wherever it touches, making the spark that connects two life forces.

Mantak Chia

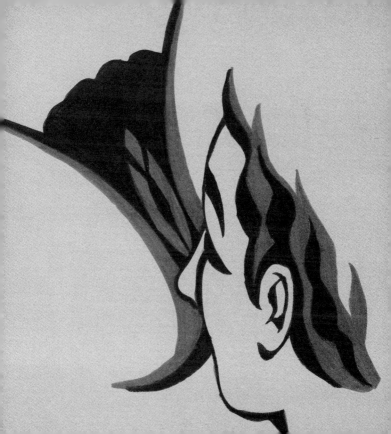

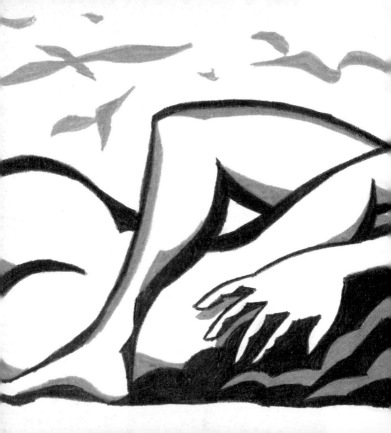

Taoists say that the exchange of vital essences generated in deep kissing helps harmonize the yin and yang forces within us. They even have a name for the saliva produced by a sexually aroused woman—"jade spring"— and urge men to sup this precious essence eagerly from their lover's mouth in the interests of health and harmony.

When kissing,
neither give nor
receive, but
become the kiss.

Merge into the dance
of hardness and
softness, yang and
yin, as your tongues
dart and retreat,
explore and yield.

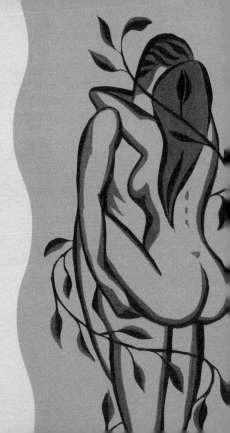

Through kissing we can bring our male and female energies into balance, playing with active and passive roles as each tongue enters the mouth of the other.

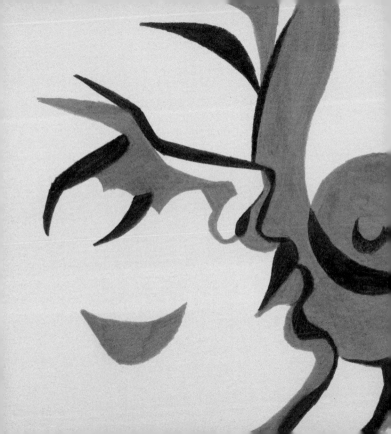

Try exploring your lover's entire body using just your mouth and tongue. It takes longer than you think!

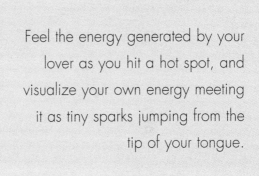

Feel the energy generated by your lover as you hit a hot spot, and visualize your own energy meeting it as tiny sparks jumping from the tip of your tongue.

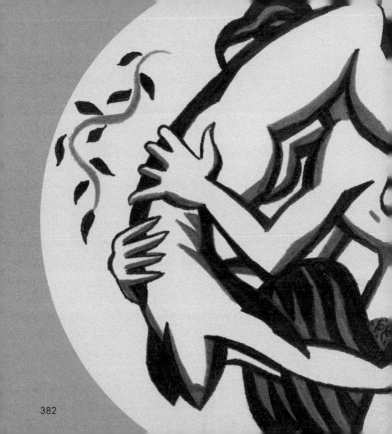

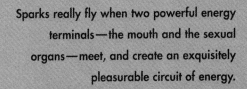

Sparks really fly when two powerful energy terminals—the mouth and the sexual organs—meet, and create an exquisitely pleasurable circuit of energy.

For its quick arousal of kundalini energy, and magical mix of love-juices and saliva, Tantrics view oral sex as a path to enlightenment!

As the vagina—or yoni—is honored as the sacred gateway to life in the Tantric tradition, pleasuring a woman's yoni with mouth and tongue, to bring her desire to the boil, is regarded as an essential part of lovemaking and an act of deep love and respect.

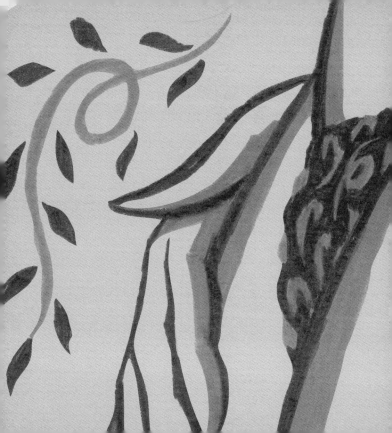

Not from bamboo or stone, not played on strings,

This is the song of an instrument that lives,

That makes the emerald tassels quiver,

Who can say what the tune is, or the key?

The red lips open wide,

The slender fingers play their part daintily.

Deep in, deep out; their hearts grow wild with passion.

There are no words to tell of the ecstasy that thrills.

The Golden Lotus

The ancient Taoists called orally pleasuring a man "playing the jade flute." Women were advised to approach the "flute" with awe and reverence, and to use their mouth as a second yoni, kissing, licking, and sucking with gentleness and enthusiasm.

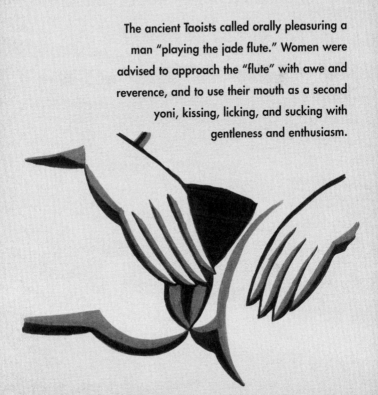

The "69" position is known as "the crow" in the Kama Sutra, and is a potent sexual posture in the Tantric tradition.

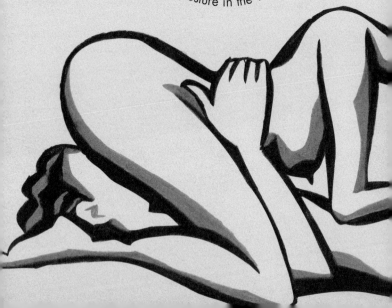

Mutual oral pleasuring is powerfully energizing, but the excitement can make it hard for both partners to bring full awareness into play. It may also be difficult to find a position comfortable enough for you both to remain in long enough to get the energy flowing. Don't be disheartened if the position doesn't work for you; it's far better to concentrate your focus and attention on bringing the greatest pleasure to each other in turn.

It is the pleasure of the bee to gather honey of the flower, but it is also the pleasure of the flower to yield its honey to the bee. For to the bee a flower is a fountain of life and to the flower a bee is a messenger of love, and to both, bee and flower, the giving and the receiving of pleasure is a need and an ecstasy.

Kahlil Gibran

THERE IS AN ART TO GIVING PLEASURE, BUT THERE IS ALSO AN ART TO RECEIVING PLEASURE. NEGLECT NEITHER.

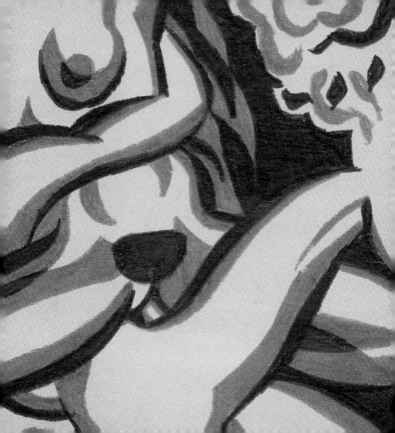

The Inuit people call sex "making laughter together."

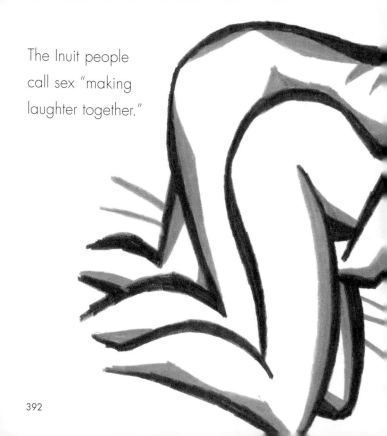

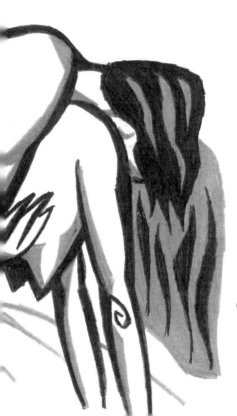

Don't forget to awaken your sense of humor with your sexuality!

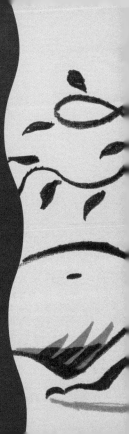

Spiritual sex is joyful, surprising, and childlike in its attitude of open-heartedness.

Let go into that joyful simplicity, and let foreplay become foreplayfulness.

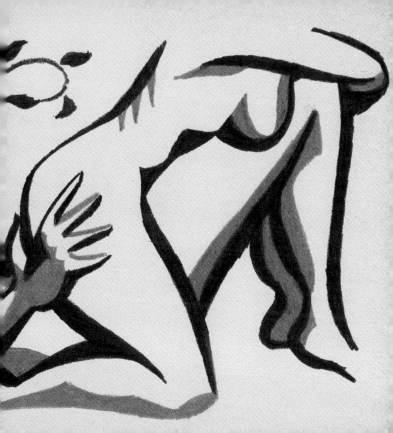

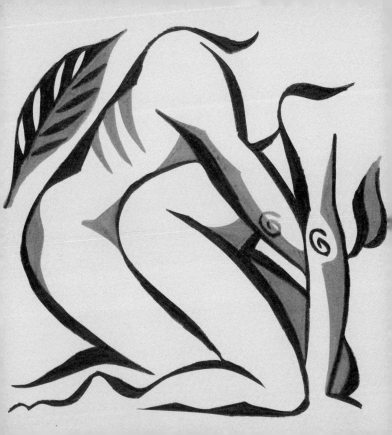

It is fun to mimic animals like dogs, deer, and goats, copying their movements and cries, to attack abruptly like the horse or arch your back like two voluptuous cats.

Kama Sutra

Be wild animals, or Tarzan and Jane in the jungle; play kiss-chase; perform a striptease; try tickling; roll about on the floor like children; decorate each other with body paints; let your guard down and simply laugh together.

Dance wildly, passionately, erotically, with or for your lover, expressing your desire and intent with every movement of your body.

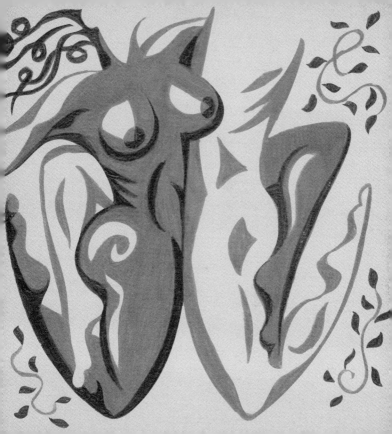

Try mystic dancing, mirroring each other's natural movements to create a harmonious mood. Express your sensuality and connection through your dance, honoring the divine in your partner with sensual, creative gestures.

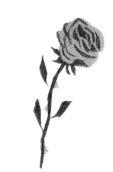

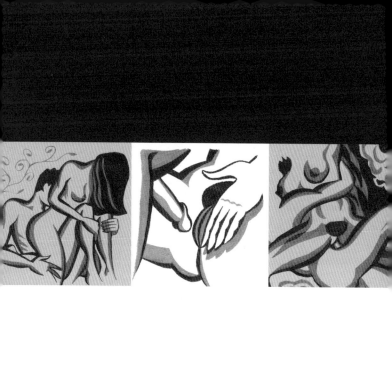

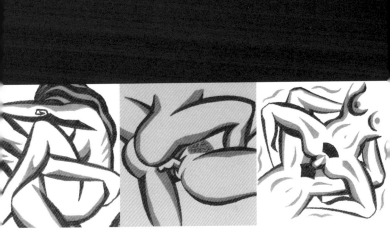

8 COSMIC **UNION**

In cosmic union we go back to our origins, to the very source of creation. We become one—with ourselves, with our lover, and with the divine. In the bliss of union we are able to touch something deeper than ourselves, to go beyond everyday reality and consciousness, and tap into the eternal cycle of creation.

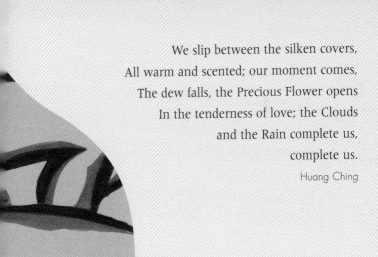

We slip between the silken covers,
All warm and scented; our moment comes,
The dew falls, the Precious Flower opens
In the tenderness of love; the Clouds
and the Rain complete us,
complete us.

Huang Ching

Male belongs to Yang.

Yang's uniqueness is that he gets
aroused quickly.

But he quickly retreats.

Female belongs to Yin.

Yin's uniqueness is that she is slower
to be aroused.

But she is also slow to retreat.

Wu Hsien

The ancient Taoist masters likened male yang energy to fire because it is easily ignited and doused. Female yin energy is said to be like water—women are slower to bring to a boil and take longer to cool down.

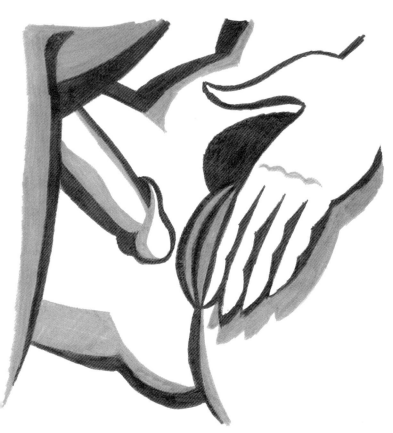

Because of the differences between yin and yang energy, the Taoists taught that men need to ensure that their lover is aroused almost to boiling point before sex can take place.

This is still good advice for lovers today. In being quick to rush into the action, it is easy to forget about the pleasures of anticipation.

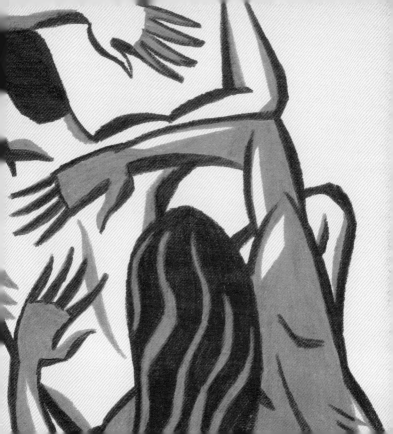

Play with the mounting sexual tension between you and within you, and let it reach almost unbearable levels before you even begin to make love.

Slowly awaken your senses to each other, and let the excitement build to bursting point—get to the edge and then linger just that little bit longer...

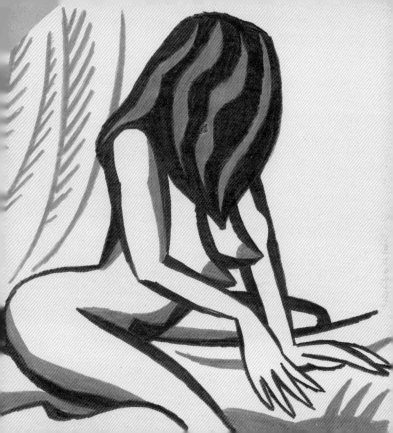

THE *KAMA SUTRA* AND OTHER ANCIENT SEX MANUALS SHOW COUPLES IN EXTRAORDINARY SEXUAL POSITIONS, BUT YOU DON'T HAVE TO GET INTO THE LOTUS POSITION TO TRANSFORM YOUR LOVEMAKING INTO A SOURCE OF SACRED BLISS.

The sexual postures outlined in Tantric texts are designed to create cosmic oneness— they help us unify male and female energies, and allow us to experience pure harmony in lovemaking by working with the flow of subtle energy within the body.

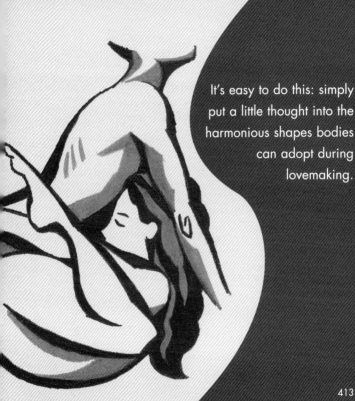

It's easy to do this: simply put a little thought into the harmonious shapes bodies can adopt during lovemaking.

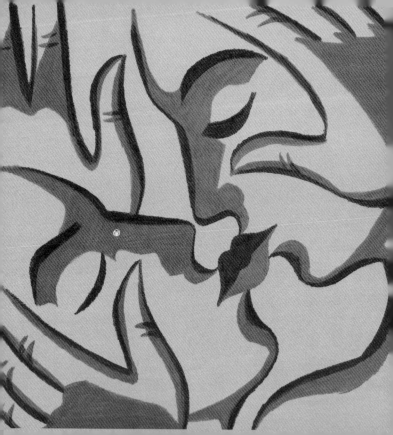

From the Tibetan tradition comes yab-yum, a loving, peaceful posture that represents the union of the male and female principles.

The man sits cross-legged while his lover is astride him in his lap, legs wrapped around his waist. This intimate position is perfect for eye-gazing, and creates a circuit of sexual energy between the two intertwined bodies.

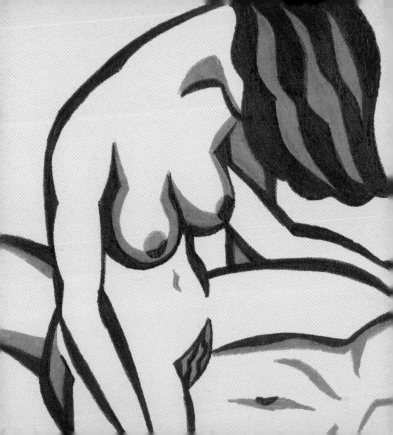

THE "WOMAN-ON-TOP" POSITION IS A TRADITIONAL TANTRIC POSTURE THAT OFFERS HER CONTROL OVER THE DEPTH OF PENETRATION, PACE, AND FLOW OF ENERGY.

While moving or still in the position, visualize pulling your lover's energy upward, through your root chakra (see page 88) and up your spine; then let the energy flow back to your lover down your arms and through your palms, deep into his body.

The kamachakra—wheel of kama—
is a classic Tantric position for resonating
energy. (In Sanskrit, kama means love,
pleasure, or sensual gratification.)

Start off in yab-yum (see page 415), then
stretch out your arms, part your legs, and
place your hands on each other's shoulders.
As you lean backward, your arms and legs
form the spokes of a wheel.

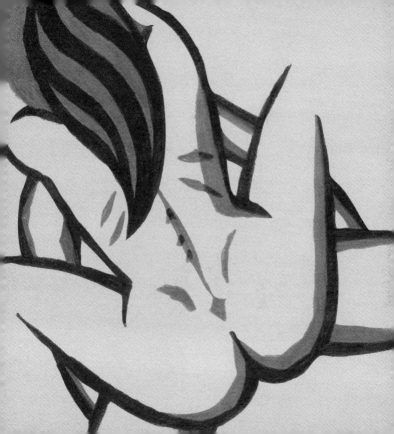

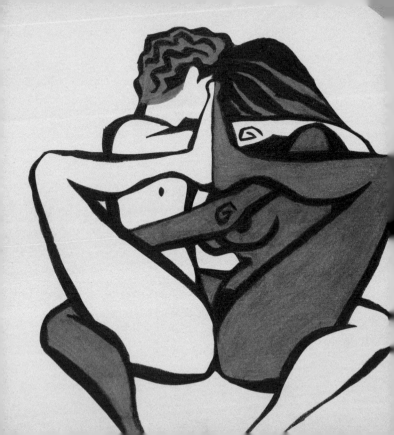

MATCH SIMILAR PARTS OF YOUR
BODIES—MOUTH TO MOUTH,
FOREHEAD TO FOREHEAD, PALM
TO PALM—TO HARMONIZE
YOUR ENERGY.

MATCH DISSIMILAR PARTS OF
YOUR BODIES—AS IN THE
"69" POSITION DURING ORAL
SEX—TO STIMULATE ENERGY.

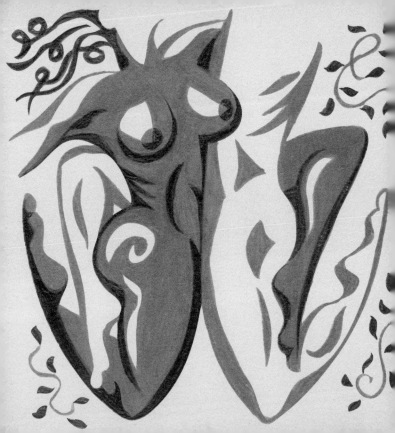

Think about your hands and feet—when touching, they can channel energy that would otherwise flow outward and be lost.

A wonderful way to experience this circuit is for the woman to lower herself onto her lover, who is sitting with his legs wide apart. She lies back between his legs, and keeps her own outstretched on either side of his body. Each partner is able to reach out and hold the feet of the other, while eye-gazing (see page 245) and breathing in tune with each other (see page 319).

There is a way of breathing
that's a shame and suffocation.
And there's another way of expiring,
a love-breath that lets you open infinitely.

Rumi

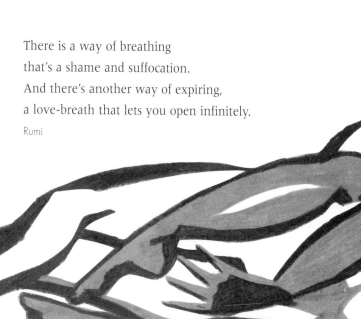

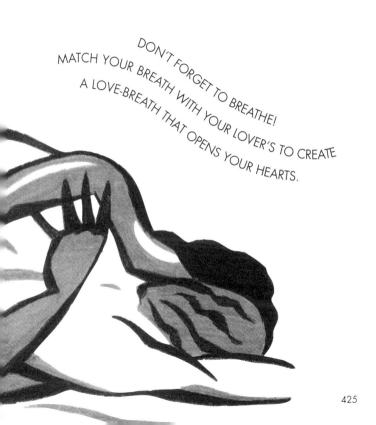

DON'T FORGET TO BREATHE!
MATCH YOUR BREATH WITH YOUR LOVER'S TO CREATE
A LOVE-BREATH THAT OPENS YOUR HEARTS.

425

THE BREATH IS A POWERFUL TOOL
FOR CIRCULATING ENERGY WITHIN
AND BETWEEN YOU.

Try connecting an energy
center, such as the heart
or third-eye chakra (see
pages 95 and 99) to your
lover's. As you inhale,
visualize energy leaving
your lover and entering
that energy center in
you. As you exhale, feel
the energy flowing out
from you and into your
lover's energy center.

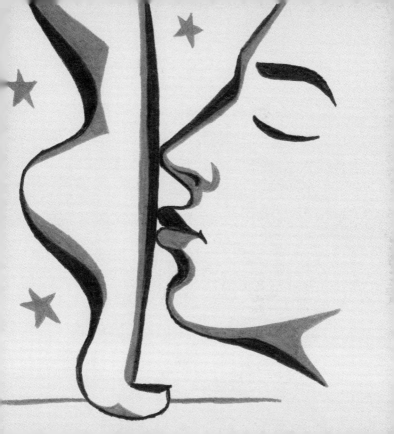

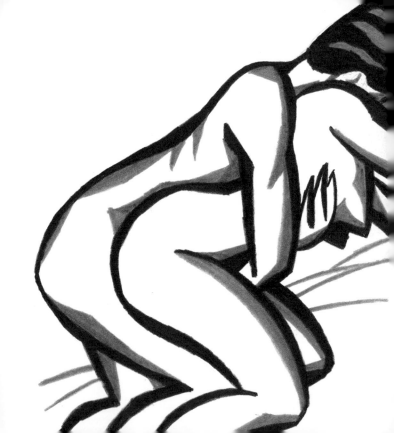

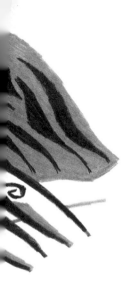

Explore different energy centers, and feel how the energy between you shifts and flows as you make contact with different parts of your bodies, and breathe as one or separately.

As you move together, you create your own erotic dance, your circle of love. Can you tell where you end and your lover begins?

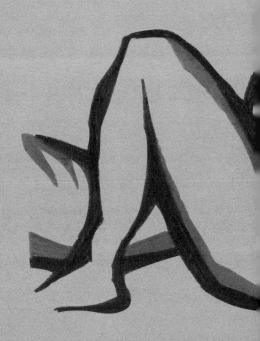

Try different postures, different rhythms; feel where they take you, then let go of them. Don't get hung up on technique. Focus on the essence, not the form.

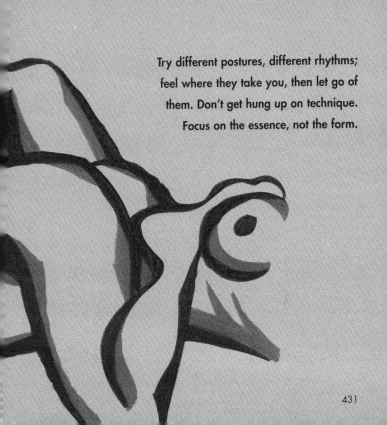

IN SPIRITUAL SEX, WE BRING AWARENESS
TO LOVEMAKING, NOT MANUALS OR
LISTS OF POSITIONS.

Coming to love with honest passion and
a meditative mind relieves you from the
need to be "exotic"—even the humble
missionary position creates a powerful
circuit of energy, with its matching of
similar body parts, and potential for
eye-gazing and deep erotic kissing.

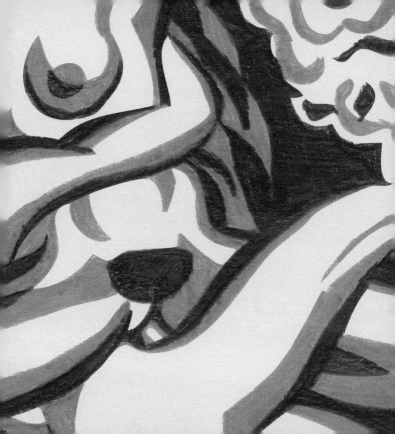

Deep and shallow, slow and swift, direct and slanting thrusts, are by no means all uniform and each has its own distinctive effect and characteristics. A slow thrust should resemble the jerking movement of a carp toying with the hook; a swift thrust that of the flight of the birds against the wind. Inserting and withdrawing, moving upward and downward, from left to right, interspaced intervals or in quick succession, and all these should be coordinated.

Seventh-century Taoist physician Li T'ung Hsuan

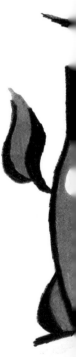

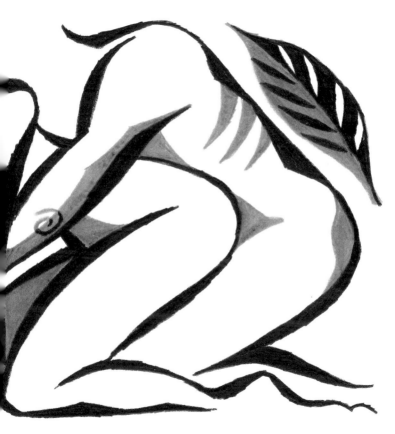

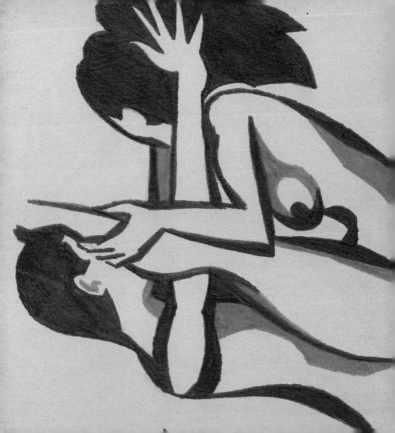

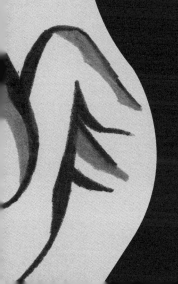

The Taoists favored varied thrusting rhythms in lovemaking, changing the style, pace, and number. This was partly to prevent tedium developing during very long Taoist lovemaking sessions!

Nine shallow, one deep is the classic Taoist thrusting method. With gentle and loving strokes, only the head of the lingam enters the yoni for nine thrusts, followed by one thrust of the entire lingam—tantalizing and satisfying for both partners.

437

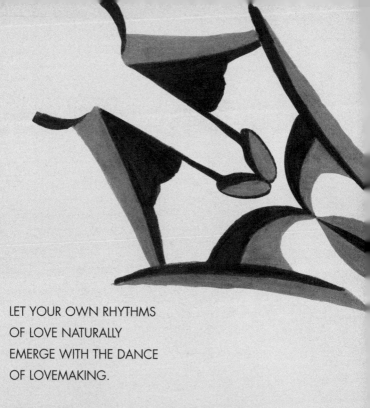

LET YOUR OWN RHYTHMS
OF LOVE NATURALLY
EMERGE WITH THE DANCE
OF LOVEMAKING.

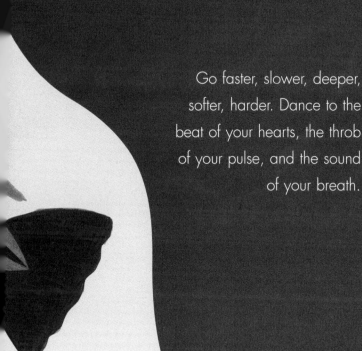

Go faster, slower, deeper, softer, harder. Dance to the beat of your hearts, the throb of your pulse, and the sound of your breath.

**In any rhythm, the space between the beat
is as important as the beat itself.**

Take a pause amid the passion for a moment
of peaceful intimacy. Feel the energy swirling
around you, and appreciate the touch of
your intertwined bodies and the sense of
peace and oneness.

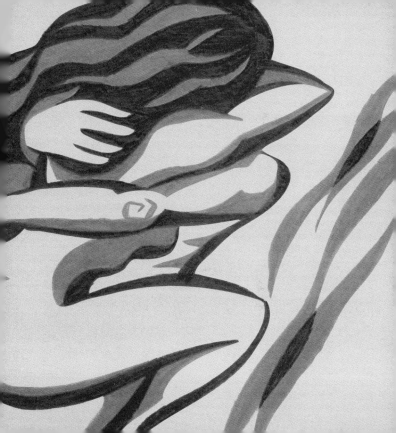

A total orgasm of the body and mind might
be described as a showering of nectar from the head,
running down your insides like a springtime shower.
It is unmistakable, a wave of subtle chi energy that
opens up hidden powers of feeling. You feel like a
newborn baby, only adult and conscious.

Mantak Chia

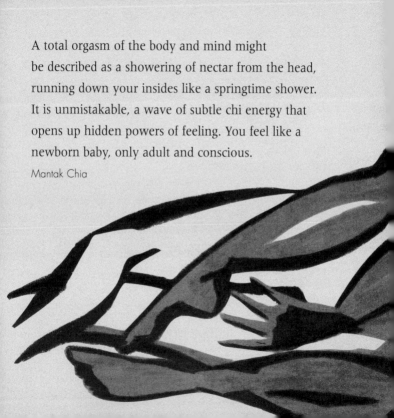

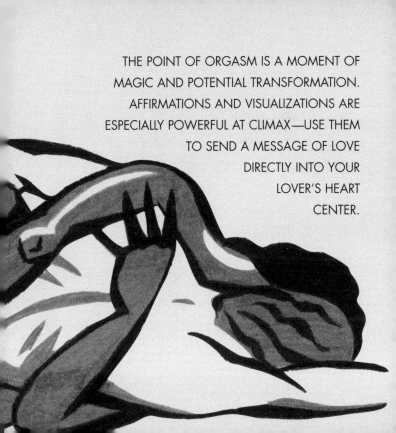

THE POINT OF ORGASM IS A MOMENT OF
MAGIC AND POTENTIAL TRANSFORMATION.
AFFIRMATIONS AND VISUALIZATIONS ARE
ESPECIALLY POWERFUL AT CLIMAX—USE THEM
TO SEND A MESSAGE OF LOVE
DIRECTLY INTO YOUR
LOVER'S HEART
CENTER.

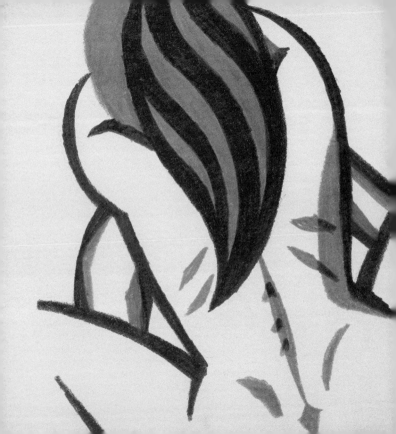

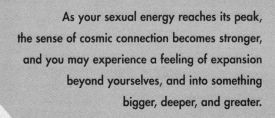

As your sexual energy reaches its peak,
the sense of cosmic connection becomes stronger,
and you may experience a feeling of expansion
beyond yourselves, and into something
bigger, deeper, and greater.

LET GO INTO THAT RELEASE,
AND SINK INTO YOUR RETURN
TO THE ULTIMATE SOURCE.

Losing yourself in the sensations of lovemaking, find yourself at one with yourself, your lover, and the creative spirit of the universe.

Playing with the hardness and softness, the tension and release, see yourself as part of the cosmic interplay of yin and yang.

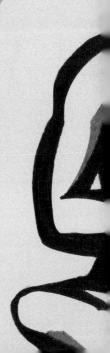

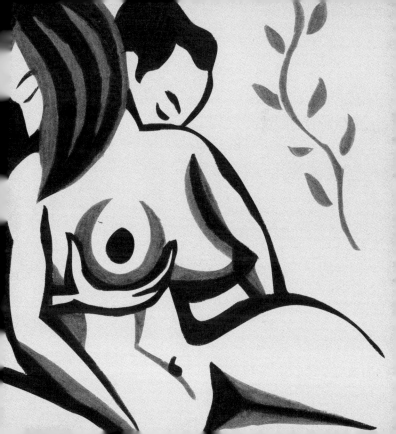

After release, stay together for a few moments longer. This is a time of powerful exchange of yin and yang essence between you, and it offers a space for renewal and awakening.

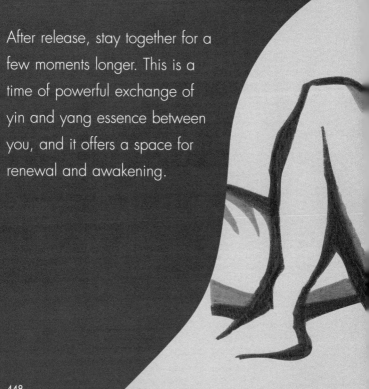

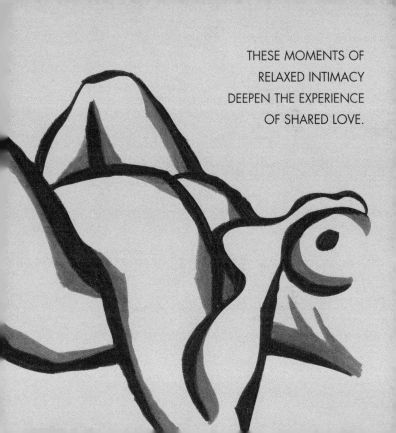

THESE MOMENTS OF
RELAXED INTIMACY
DEEPEN THE EXPERIENCE
OF SHARED LOVE.

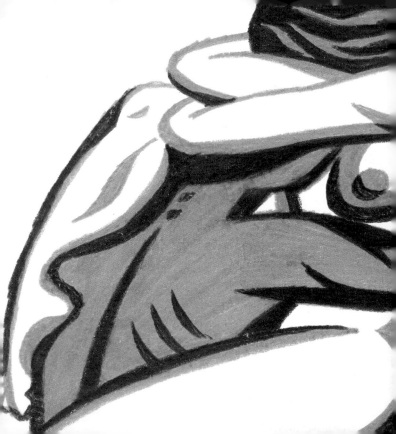

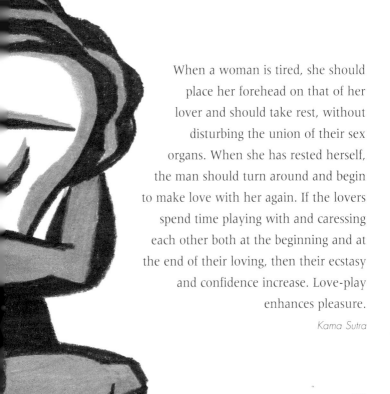

When a woman is tired, she should place her forehead on that of her lover and should take rest, without disturbing the union of their sex organs. When she has rested herself, the man should turn around and begin to make love with her again. If the lovers spend time playing with and caressing each other both at the beginning and at the end of their loving, then their ecstasy and confidence increase. Love-play enhances pleasure.

Kama Sutra

Keep the connection alive as you bathe in the afterglow of your loving union, and feel the waves of tingling post-orgasmic energy rippling through and between you.

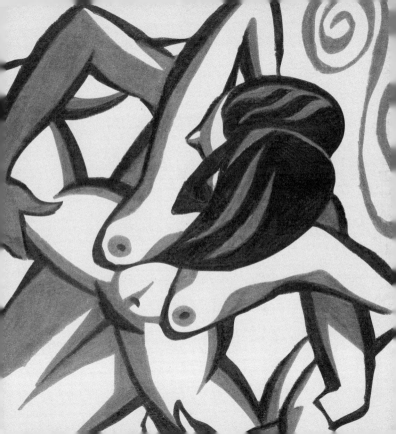

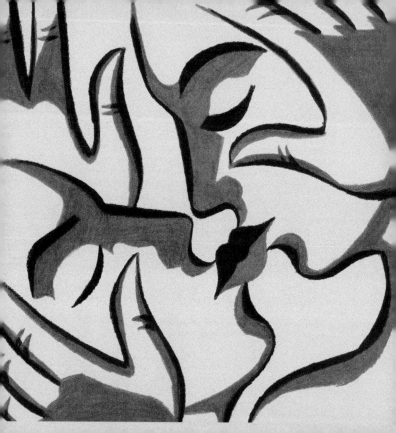

As your heart connection is fully open, this is a special time together—be gentle with yourself and your lover. Of course, lying intertwined, gently stroking and cuddling, may eventually lead you to want to start over—afterplay merging into foreplay in one delicious circle of pleasure.

Sacred sex is a journey that doesn't end at orgasm.

The spiritual connection we experience through sexual intimacy continues long after the lovemaking itself is over. It acts as a beacon shedding light on the world, suggesting new ways to interact with those around us.

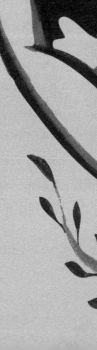

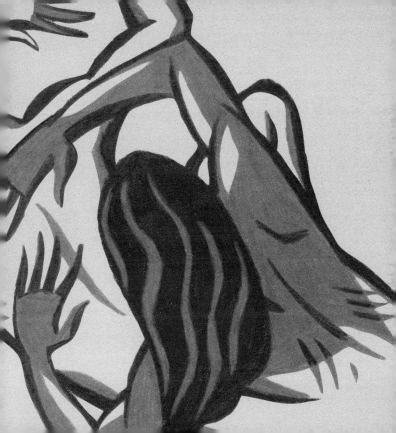

The sense of expansion we discover in spiritual sex can be extended into every part of life.

When we say "Yes" to life, to the full potential of the senses and of body, mind, and spirit, we open up possibilities beyond our wildest imaginings.

The love we make showers love on the world—take your love out into the world and see where it takes you.

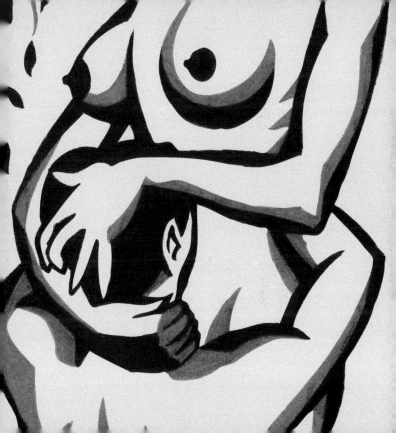

A road might end at a single house,
but it's not love's road.

Love is a river.
Drink from it.

Rumi

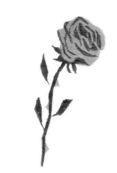

Bibliography

Aldred, Caroline. *Divine Sex*. Carroll and Brown, London, 2000.

Anand, Margo. *The Art of Sexual Ecstasy*. Tarcher, Putnam, Los Angeles, CA, 1989.

Anand, Margo. *The Art of Sexual Magic*. Piatkus, London, 1995.

Barefoot Doctor. *Barefoot Doctor's Handbook for Modern Lovers*. Piatkus, London, 2000.

Burton, Sir Richard and Arbuthnot, F F. *Kama Sutra of Vatsyayana*. Thorsons, London, 1999.

Chia, Mantak and Maneewan. *Taoist Secrets of Love: cultivating male sexual energy*. Aurora Press, Santa Fe, NM, 1984.

Chia, Mantak and Maneewan. *Healing Love through the Tao: cultivating female sexual energy*. Healing Tao Books, Santa Fe, NM, 1986.

Chia, Mantak and Maneewan, and Carlton Abrams, Douglas and Rachel. *Multi-Orgasmic Couple*. Thorsons, London, 2000.

Chang, Jolan. *The Tao of Love and Sex*. Wildwood, Aldershot, Hampshire, 1997.

Doniger, Wendy and Kakar, Sudhir. *Kamasutra*. Oxford University Press, Oxford, 2002.

Douglas, Nik and Slinger, Penny. *Sexual Secrets: the alchemy of ecstasy*. Destiny Books, Rochester, VM, 2000.

Douglas, Nik. *Spiritual Sex*. Pocket Books, New York, 1997.

Johnston, Bonnie L and Schuerman, Peter L. *Sex, Magick and Spirit*. Llewellyn, 1998.

Lorius, Cassandra. *Tantric Sex: making love last*. Thorsons, London, 1999.

Ma Anand Sarita and Swami Anand Geho. *Tantric Love*. Gaia Books, London, 2001.

Muir, Charles and Caroline. *Tantra, the Art of Conscious Loving*. Mercury House, San Francisco, CA, 1989.

Ramsdale, David and Ellen. *Sexual Energy Ecstasy*. Bantam, New York, NY, 1985.

Reid, Daniel. *The Tao of Health, Sex and Longevity*. Simon and Schuster, London, 1989.

Shaw, Miranda. *Passionate Enlightenment: women in tantric Buddhism*. Princeton, Princeton, NJ, 1994.

Toshio Sudo, Philip. *Zen Sex*. HarperSanFrancisco, San Francisco, CA, 2000.

With love and thanks to D

Acknowledgements

The author and the publisher wish to thank the following for granting permission to use extracts from their books in *Spiritual Sex*:

p.78, p.118, p.173, p.182, p.186, p.189, p.217, p.224, p.284, p.294, p.302, and p.310: Douglas, Nik; *Spiritual Sex* (Pocket Books, New York, 1997). Reprinted by permission of Inner Traditions.

p.29, p.64, p.135, p.176, p.263, p.270, p.343, and p.344: Shaw, Miranda; *Passionate Enlightenment: Women in Tantric Buddhism*. Copyright © 1994 by Princeton University Press. Reprinted by permission of Princeton University Press.

Every effort has been made to trace and contact current copyright holders. Any omission is unintentional, and the publisher would be pleased to hear from any copyright holders not acknowledged above.

Michelle Pauli is a researcher and writer on spirituality and alternative religion, with an MSc from the London School of Economics. She gained an extensive knowledge of spiritual practice and experience from her work with Inform, a charity that provides objective information about new religious movements to academics and the media.

Michelle is the author of *Sex with Spirit* (Red Wheel/Weiser, 2002), and co-author of *In Search of the Ultimate High: Spiritual Experience Through Psychoactives* (Rider Books, Random House, London, 2000). She has also contributed to a volume on dance culture, *Party Politics* (Verso, London, 2002). As a freelance journalist, she writes for many publications and websites. She lives in London, England.

Published by MQ Publications Limited
12 The Ivories, 6–8 Northampton Street
London N1 2HY
Tel: 020 7359 2244   Fax: 020 7359 1616
email: mail@mqpublications.com

Editor: Salima Hirani
Design: Philippa Jarvis
Illustrations: Alan Adler

ISBN: 1–84072–420–X

1 3 5 7 9 0 8 6 4 2

Printed and bound in Hong Kong